② 12.50

CEFN COED
MEDICAL
KT-461-744

Self-assessment for Psychiatry Examinations

Cefn Coed Library
Z003009

SWANSEA PSYCHIATRIC EDUCATION
LIBRARY

DATE DUE

22/3/06		
4/11/13		

Demco No. 62-0549

Self-assessment for Psychiatry Examinations

Basant K. Puri
MA MB BChir
Senior Research Associate in Neuroscience, Peterhouse, Cambridge; Honorary Registrar, University of Cambridge Department of Psychiatry

Gregory J. Weppner
MB BS MRCPsych
Senior Registrar in Psychiatry, Department of Psychological Medicine, University of Wales, Heath Park, Cardiff

Foreword by
Professor E. S. Paykel
MD FRCP FRCPsych
Professor of Psychiatry, University of Cambridge

SWANSEA PSYCHIATRIC EDUCATION LIBRARY

Churchill Livingstone

EDINBURGH LONDON MELBOURNE AND NEW YORK 1989

CHURCHILL LIVINGSTONE
Medical Division of Longman Group UK Limited

Distributed in the United States of America by Churchill
Livingstone Inc., 1560 Broadway, New York, N.Y. 10036,
and by associated companies, branches and
representatives throughout the world.

© Longman Group UK Limited 1989

All rights reserved. No part of this publication may be
reproduced, stored in a retrieval system, or transmitted
in any form or by any means, electronic, mechanical,
photocopying, recording or otherwise, without either the
prior written permission of the publishers (Churchill
Livingstone, Robert Stevenson House, 1–3 Baxter's
Place, Leith Walk, Edinburgh EH1 3AF), or a licence
permitting restricted copying in the United Kingdom
issued by the Copyright Licensing Agency Ltd, 33–34
Alfred Place, London, WC1E 7DP.

First published 1989

ISBN 0-443-04171-7

British Library Cataloguing in Publication Data
Puri, Basant K.
    Self-assessment for psychiatry examinations
    1. Medicine. Psychiatry. Questions &
    answers
    I. Title   II. Weppner, Greig J.
    616.89'0076

Library of Congress Cataloging in Publication Data
Puri, Basant K.
    Self-assessment for psychiatry examinations.
    1. Psychiatry — Examinations, questions, etc.
I. Weppner, Grieg J. II. Title. [DNLM: 1. Psychiatry —
examination questions. WM 18 P985s]
RC457.P87 1989   616.89'0076   88-35348

Produced by Longman Singapore Publishers (Pte) Ltd.
Printed in Singapore

Preface

In 1988, for the first time in its history, major changes have taken place in both the syllabus and the structure of the MRCPsych Part II (Membership) Examination. The main changes have involved the introduction of a Short Answer Question Paper (50% Basic Sciences and 50% Clinical Topics) and also a second Multiple Choice Paper on Sciences Basic to Psychiatry. This book consists of six multiple choice question papers and three short answer question papers which follow exactly the new MRCPsych Examination format and which cover the entire new expanded syllabus. Explanations, where required, are given for the answers. Furthermore, full references are provided for each answer.

This book covers thoroughly the new examination syllabus, with questions and full answers and references on the following areas: Psychology; Ethology; Neurophysiology; Neurochemistry; Clinical Pharmacology; Social Studies; Genetics; Epidemiology; Medical Statistics; Psychometrics; Research Methods; Aspects of General Medicine Applied to Psychiatry; the Assessment and Management of Psychiatric Disorders in Children (including clinical and community aspects); the Assessment and Management of Psychiatric Disorders in Adults (including clinical and community aspects); the Assessment and Management of Psychiatric Disorders in Adults (including clinical and community aspects); the Assessment and Management of Psychiatric Disorders in the Elderly (including clinical and community aspects); the Psychiatry of Mental Handicap; Forensic Psychiatry; Psychotherapy; Substance Abuse; Sexual Problems; Aspects of Epidemiology related to Clinical Psychiatry; and the History of Psychiatry.

Candidates for the new examination will find these model papers and answers of great help in their revision. It is recommended that each paper be answered under Examination conditions, as follows:

Sciences Basic to Psychiatry MCQ Paper — $1\frac{1}{2}$ hours (50 questions)
Clinical Topics MCQ Paper — $1\frac{1}{2}$ hours (50 questions)
Short Answer Question Paper — $1\frac{1}{2}$ hours (20 questions)

Some candidates sell themselves short by answering only the stems to which they are certain of the answers. Candidates rarely obtain a perfect score even if they do this. At best they may obtain a lower mark than they otherwise would. At worst they may answer less than the number required to pass. Many candidates may be good at guessing or may actually know more than they think they do. One means of testing this hypothesis in a personal way is to answer one of the MCQ papers in this book in the following manner. Initially go through the paper very quickly without pondering on the question, placing a T or F beside every stem. Then with a different coloured pen, answer them at the rate you would in the examination. Answer all the questions. At the same time place a 1, 2 or 3 beside each answer using the following method:

1 — if you are certain that your answer is correct
2 — for a guess that you feel has a greater than 50% chance of being correct
3 — if you are certain you do not know the answer

It is then a simple matter to compare the percentage of correct answers in each of the categories, and then decide on your own MCQ strategy.

The definitions of the words used in the stems of the multiple choice questions have been based on those given by Dr. John Anderson in his excellent book *The Multiple Choice Question in Medicine*[1]. The syllabus used as the basis of the multiple choice questions and the short answer questions is that given in the Eighth Revision of the *General Information and Regulations for the MRCPsych Examination*.

We should like to thank the staff at Churchill Livingstone for their help and encouragement during the process of preparing this book for press.

Lastly, we should also like to express our thanks to Professor E. S. Paykel for his very helpful advice and his generosity in kindly providing a Foreword.

Cambridge   B.K.P.
Cardiff   ·   G.J.W.
1989

1. Anderson J 1982 The Multiple Choice Question in Medicine, 2nd edn. Pitman Books Ltd, London
2. The Royal College of Psychiatrists 1987 General information and regulations for the MRCPsych examinations, 8th revision. The Royal College of Psychiatrists, London

Foreword

Multiple choice questions are a relatively recent arrival in British examinations and not all candidates find their approach easy. The fine ambiguities of wording which can creep into even the best constructed of questions present particular problems for the overseas candidate whose first language is not English, and who has not been able to develop fully an idiomatic intuition for what might have been in the examiner's mind.

It is healthy to be reminded that such questions do not merely provide a hurdle to be overcome, but can provide a useful way of learning. Revising in this way may familiarize with exam technique at the same time as it tests knowledge.

The authors of this volume start from a particular vantage point. They are able young psychiatrists, close enough to the recent experience of learning and being examined in which they seek to assist others. Their book is impressive in its comprehensive factual cover and well targeted on a specific examination which forms an important qualification in the professional training of young British psychiatrists today. I am pleased to be able to commend and support it.

Cambridge, 1989   E. S. Paykel

Contents

Questions

Paper 1: MULTIPLE CHOICE QUESTIONS ON BASIC SCIENCES

1.1 An average 30-week-old child
- **A** can stand with slight support
- **B** is able to speak single words
- **C** has begun to develop grasping and manipulation
- **D** is beginning to develop ocular control
- **E** has developed gender identity.

1.2 The following are associated with Piaget's concept of cognitive development
- **A** urethral eroticism
- **B** precausal reasoning
- **C** trust versus mistrust
- **D** authoritarian morality
- **E** anal retention.

1.3 The following are associated with Margaret Mahler
- **A** practising period
- **B** rapprochement
- **C** animism
- **D** differentiation
- **E** consolidation.

1.4 Features of dysfunction of the frontal lobe include
- **A** finger agnosia
- **B** alexia
- **C** polydipsia
- **D** cortical sensory loss
- **E** increased initiative.

1.5 The Repertory Grid test
- **A** is a semi-standardized method of interviewing
- **B** can only be used with patients with thought disorder
- **C** is associated with the Personal Construct Theory
- **D** is useful in assessing organic deterioration
- **E** is based on the theory of Kelly.

1.6   Flooding

   A   is an aversion therapy
   B   is the most effective treatment of agoraphobia
   C   is an effective treatment of animal phobias
   D   can involve implosive therapy
   E   entails the unpredictable presentation of stimuli.

1.7   Fast activity on the EEG is caused by

   A   chlorpromazine
   B   amitriptyline
   C   amylobarbitone
   D   lithium carbonate
   E   diazepam.

1.8   In maternally deprived monkeys, it is found that

   A   as they are developing, they appear to enjoy being with
        each other
   B   as adults they hiss and spit at intruders to their cages
   C   adult females generally do not present sexually to normal
        adult males
   D   adult males rarely copulate normally with normal adult
        females
   E   adult females in their own turn make poor mothers.

**1.9   The following neurotransmitters are believed to be involved in
the neurochemistry of sleep**

   A   substance P
   B   dopamine
   C   serotonin
   D   noradrenaline
   E   acetylcholine.

1.10   Sympathetic ganglia may be

   A   stimulated by smoking cigarettes
   B   blocked by α-methyldopa
   C   blocked by muscarine
   D   stimulated by noradrenaline
   E   blocked by hexamethonium.

**1.11   The actions of the neurotransmitter acetylcholine at nerve
endings can be limited by**

   A   pseudocholinesterase
   B   hydrolysis
   C   anticholinesterases
   D   being broken down to acetic acid and choline
   E β-receptor antagonists.

1.12 The following are intermediates in the biosynthesis of adrenaline

A dopa
B tryptophan
C noradrenaline
D phenylethylamine
E tyrosine.

1.13 The following hormones are directly under the control of the hypothalamus

A thyroxine
B oxytocin
C follicle-stimulating hormone
D corticotrophin
E somatotrophin.

1.14 The basal ganglia include the following

A cingulate gyrus
B caudate
C globus pallidus
D mamillary body
E putamen.

1.15 Constriction of the pupils with accommodation involves the following structures

A cerebral cortex
B optic tracts
C third nerve nuclei
D lateral geniculate nuclei
E optic nerves.

1.16 The following structures lie within the diencephalon

A cerebellum
B basal ganglia
C pons
D thalamus
E hypothalamus.

1.17 Dopamine is

A produced from tryptophan
B found mainly in raphé neurones
C metabolized to homovanillic acid
D metabolized by monoamine oxidase
E released in a calcium-dependent process in the central nervous system.

1.18 The following are intermediates in the biosynthesis of serotonin

A   histidine
B   hydroxyhistamine
C   hydroxytryptamine
D   tyrosine
E   hyroxyindolacetic acid.

1.19 Neurotransmitter biosynthesis occurs at the following sites

A   5-hydroxytryptamine: medulla
B   dopamine: locus coeruleus
C   endorphins: hypothalamus
D   adrenaline: raphé nuclei
E   noradrenaline: motor cortex.

1.20 Opioid kappa receptors are probably involved in

A   miosis
B   supraspinal inhibition of pain responses
C   respiratory stimulation
D   spinal analgesia
E   sedation.

1.21 Side-effects of chlorpromazine include

A   failure of ejaculation
B   hypothermia
C   gynaecomastia
D   thrombocytopenia
E   abnormal T-waves on the ECG.

1.22 The following are examples of dystonia

A   lead-pipe rigidity
B   torticollis
C   opisthotonus
D   tongue contraction
E   trismus.

1.23 The following substances are known to enhance the affinity of GABA receptor sites for GABA

A   propranolol
B   methadone
C   lorazepam
D   ethanol
E   amylobarbitone.

1.24 Compared with amitriptyline, mianserin is more likely to cause

A haematological reactions
B anticholinergic effects
C hepatic reactions
D cardiovascular reactions.
E hypertensive crisis.

1.25 Amphetamines may be used in treating

A anorexia
B depression
C narcolepsy
D personality disorder
E hyperkinetic syndrome.

1.26 Drugs that interact dangerously with monoamine oxidase inhibitors include

A propranolol
B methyldopa
C morphine
D ephedrine nasal drops
E pemoline.

1.27 Institutional neurosis

A was a term first used by Wing
B has ability to plan for the future as a common feature
C is dependent on the original illness when it occurs in hospital
D is often characterized by low self-esteem
E is often preventable.

1.28 Mortification processes

A may lead to institutionalization
B may cause rebellion against staff
C are secondary handicaps
D were first described by Belknap
E may cause withdrawal into fantasy life.

1.29 In the US/UK Diagnostic Project (Cooper et al 1972), patients were sometimes diagnosed as suffering from schizophrenia in New York, when in London they were regarded as having

A schizophrenia
B mania
C depressive illness
D personality disorder
E neurotic illness.

1.30 In illness behaviour
- A the person feels ill
- B the person takes measures to prevent disease
- C activity is undertaken to define the state of health
- D activity is undertaken to discover a suitable remedy
- E activity is undertaken to detect asymptomatic disease.

1.31 The extended family is also known as
- A the conjugal family
- B the joint family
- C the consanguine family
- D the nuclear family
- E exogamy.

1.32 The present-day determinants of social class include
- A education
- B occupation
- C income
- D leisure activities
- E property ownership.

1.33 The following are recessive conditions
- A tyrosinosis
- B homocystinuria
- C Gaucher's disease
- D Wilson's disease
- E neurofibromatosis.

1.34 The following may show sex-linked inheritance
- A tuberous sclerosis
- B Hunter's syndrome
- C Hurler's syndrome
- D Oculocerebrorenal syndrome of Lowe
- E Lesch–Nyhan syndrome.

1.35 Down's syndrome
- A is more frequent with increasing maternal age
- B may be caused by trisomy of chromosome 21
- C is associated more with paternal than maternal dysfunction
- D may result from mosaicism
- E predisposes to presenility.

1.36 The following may show autosomal dominant transmission
- A Huntington's chorea
- B Marfan's syndrome
- C acute intermittent porphyria
- D tuberous sclerosis
- E hyperuricaemia.

1.37 Klinefelter's syndrome is
  A commoner in females
  B an X-linked condition
  C chromatin-positive
  D typically seen in tall thin individuals
  E associated with an increased incidence of sexual disorders.

1.38 In general medicine
  A a person can have a disease without being ill
  B a person can be ill without having a disease
  C illness can be defined as the absence of health
  D illness can be defined as the presence of suffering
  E illness can be defined in terms of pathological processes.

1.39 In psychiatry the term 'part function' as used by A. J. Lewis refers to
  A emotion
  B death
  C perception
  D memory
  E learning.

1.40 Categorical classification systems in psychiatry include
  A ICD 9
  B DSM-III R axis V
  C Eysenck's personality scales
  D Fould's classification
  E The WHO child psychiatry classificatory system (Rutter et al 1975).

1.41 It has been shown that British family doctors in general detect emotional disorders more readily in the following groups
  A homosexuals
  B women
  C widows
  D the middle-aged
  E married men.

1.42 The recorded rate of suicide in Britain increased during the following periods
  A World War I in men
  B World War I in women
  C World War II in men
  D World War II in women
  E 1932–1933 (a time of economic depression and high unemployment).

1.43   Deliberate self-harm rates are higher in
   A   older than in younger people
   B   men than in women
   C   social class I than in social class V
   D   the divorced than in the married
   E   areas of high unemployment.

1.44   In the UK, important information about the prevalence of drug dependence comes from
   A   criminal statistics
   B   employers' statistics
   C   Home Office statistics
   D   hospital admissions
   E   special surveys.

1.45   Pascal's triangle
   A   can be used when the probabilities of two events occurring are equal
   B   can be used when the probabilities of two events occurring are unequal
   C   can be used in the binomial distribution
   D   is a test of significance
   E   can be used to determine regression to the mean.

1.46   In a positively skewed unimodal distribution the
   A   standard deviation is a good measure of variability
   B   right-hand side tail is the longer one
   C   standard deviation is always less than or equal to the variance
   D   mean is greater than the mode
   E   mean is less than the median.

1.47   95% confidence limits for the mean of a large sample in a particular experiment are 1 to 5. This implies that
   A   the population mean is significantly different from zero
   B   the probability that the range 1 to 5 contains the population mean is 0.95
   C   the standard error of the mean (used to construct the confidence interval) is approximately 4
   D   the population mean is significantly different from 4.75
   E   the correlation coefficient is 0.95.

1.48 In a trial in which a single group of patients is measured
before and after using a new drug, one would expect that the
following alternative hypotheses for the observed change could
be ruled out

    A placebo effect
    B spontaneous remission
    C Hawthorne effect
    D natural illness fluctuation
    E poor clinician–patient communication.

1.49 The null hypothesis is a statement that

    A accurately predicts the results of clinical trials
    B implies p is 0.05
    C is always true
    D may be erroneously thought to be false but would always be
proven to be true if enough observations were made
    E states there is no significant difference between the
experimental and control groups.

1.50 The exact test of Fisher is

    A a test which involves the use of factorials
    B impractical for large samples
    C suitable for samples where the numbers are too small for
chi-squared
    D an exact probability test
    E used in the analysis of fourfold tables.

PAPER 2: MULTIPLE CHOICE QUESTIONS ON CLINICAL TOPICS

2.1 Recognized features of acute organic psychiatric syndromes
include

    A repetitive purposeless movements
    B disorientation in place
    C tactile hallucinations
    D ideas of reference
    E impaired registration.

2.2 Creutzfeldt–Jakob disease

    A is genetically transmitted
    B may cause extrapyramidal signs
    C is another name for kuru
    D has ataxia as a common feature
    E is characterized by intellectual deterioration.

2.3   Following a penetrating head injury, the amount of brain tissue destruction is related to the following

A   mental state after 1 year
B   neurotic symptoms
C   apathy
D   poor judgement
E   euphoria.

2.4   Recognized features of vitamin B$_{12}$ deficiency include

A   glove and stocking anaesthesia
B   depression
C   psychosis
D   optic neuritis
E   memory loss.

2.5   In co-proxamol overdosage

A   the administration of naloxone may be life-saving
B   coma may occur
C   respiratory depression may occur
D   the pupils are typically dilated
E   patients may die of acute cardiovascular collapse.

2.6   In complex partial seizures

A   seizures always arise in the temporal lobe
B   intense disturbances of emotion may occur
C   attacks typically start without an aura
D   automatisms may occur
E   consciousness is usually not impaired.

2.7   In normal-pressure hydrocephalus

A   the EEG is typically abnormal
B   there is obstruction within the ventricles
C   the gait is commonly abnormal
D   surgery may help
E   the ventricles are not enlarged.

2.8   The battered baby syndrome

A   is commonly perpetrated by a parent who was subjected to physical abuse as a child
B   is a term introduced by Kempe
C   the child may be dehydrated
D   the parents rarely deny their role
E   the child acts normally in the presence of its parents.

2.9 Neurotic disorders in childhood
A are the most frequent psychiatric disorders of childhood
B are more than twice as common in girls as in boys
C are commonly hysterical
D are commonly obsessional
E are most commonly anxiety disorders in mid-childhood.

2.10 Childhood behaviours that can be regarded as depressive equivalents include
A truancy
B running away from home
C promiscuity
D boredom
E bullying.

2.11 The term hyperkinetic syndrome, as used in Britain, includes the following features
A temper tantrums
B learning difficulties
C short episodes of motor overactivity
D mood fluctuation
E aggression.

2.12 The ICD 9 classification of personality disorders includes the following categories
A dependent
B schizotypal
C histrionic
D obsessive–compulsive
E explosive.

2.13 Types of body build described by Kretschmer include
A endomorphy
B mesomorphy
C ectomorphy
D somatotonia
E cyclothymic.

2.14 In neurotic disorders
A symptoms may persist even when the original cause has disappeared
B genetic factors are of little or no importance
C the death rate is greater than average
D stressful conditions at work are an important cause
E medication is an effective form of long-term treatment.

2.15 Agoraphobia

  A   can cause a person to remain housebound
  B   may present with palpitations
  C   is the same as social phobic neurosis
  D   may arise secondary to a depressive disorder
  E   symptoms may be reduced by the presence of a pet.

2.16 Characteristics of an obsessional personality include

  A   high moral standards
  B   rigidity in views held
  C   indecision
  D   sensitivity to criticism
  E   unexpressed feelings of resentment.

2.17 As compared with depressive disorders, features that are commoner after bereavement include

  A   numbness
  B   retardation
  C   suicidal thoughts
  D   guilt about past actions in general
  E   complaints of physical symptoms.

2.18 Regarding the concept of learned helplessness

  A   it was propounded by Bowlby
  B   it is a learning theory view of depression
  C   it suggests that depression develops when reward or punishment is no longer clearly contingent on the actions of the organism
  D   increased voluntary activity is a characteristic feature
  E   reduced food intake is a characteristic feature.

2.19 Bruxism

  A   occurs in stages I and II of sleep
  B   responds well to tricyclic antidepressant treatment
  C   tends to run in families
  D   is commoner in children
  E   may cause physical damage.

2.20 Schneider's first-rank symptoms include

  A   delusions of persecution
  B   thought withdrawal
  C   voices speaking to the person
  D   ideas of reference
  E   echolalia.

2.21 **The following categories of depressive disorder were described by Paykel after the use of cluster analysis**
   A   asthenic
   B   hostile
   C   anxious
   D   older depressive with personality disorder
   E   psychotic.

2.22 **Regarding the syndrome of benign senescent forgetfulness**
   A   the disorder is primarily one of recall
   B   it is a form of arteriosclerotic dementia
   C   it was first described by Roth
   D   there is progressive difficulty in remembering
   E   there is a significantly diminished lifespan.

2.23 **Clinical features of multi-infarct dementia include**
   A   gradual onset
   B   more common in females
   C   fits
   D   depressive symptoms
   E   stepwise progression.

2.24 **In patients being treated by psychiatrists for manic-depressive psychosis and reactive depression**
   A   the risk of dying by suicide is approximately 30 times the risk in the general population
   B   less than 10% will die by suicide if patients are followed up for life
   C   there is a decreased risk of suicide in the first 2 years following initial treatment
   D   women are at higher risk of suicide than men
   E   the young are at higher risk of suicide than the old.

2.25 **In English general medical hospital wards**
   A   acute organic syndromes are a common psychiatric disorder
   B   affective disorders are a common psychiatric disorder
   C   schizophrenia is a common psychiatric disorder
   D   alcohol-related disorders are common
   E   in the study by Maguire et al (1974) approximately half the psychiatric morbidity was not recognized by the physicians or nurses.

2.26 Findings from the studies by Rutter & Graham (1985) on children living in the Isle of Wight and an inner London borough showed the following

A   the 1-year prevalence rate of psychiatric disorder was approximately equal in boys and girls

B   the rates of all types of psychiatric disorder in the Isle of Wight were approximately twice those in an inner London borough

C   at age 14 the 1-year prevalence rate of handicapping psychiatric disorders was over 10%

D   hysteria was encountered rarely in the community

E   the 1-year prevalence rate of prepubertal depressive disorders of the adult type was over 10%.

2.27 The following are drugs that should either be avoided or used with caution in breastfeeding mothers

A   chlormethiazole

B   mianserin

C   methadone

D   lithium carbonate

E   sulpiride.

2.28 The following statements concerning phenothiazines are true

A   fluphenazine is a piperidine compound

B   piperidine compounds generally have fewer extrapyramidal side-effects than piperazine compounds

C   aliphatic compounds are generally less sedating than piperazine compounds

D   haloperidol is usually a safe phenothiazine to administer in mania

E   piperazine compounds generally have fewer anticholinergic effects than piperidine compounds.

2.29 Concerning psychosurgery, the following statements are true

A   sexual psychopathology is occasionally an indication for standard bilateral prefrontal leucotomy

B   thalamotomy is generally performed with the patient fully conscious

C   psychogenic pain is occasionally an indication for hypophysectomy

D   stereotactic anterior cingulotomy has been used to treat intractable pain

E   stereotactic limbic leucotomy is one of the main psychosurgical operations carried out in the UK.

2.30 Side-effects of ECT include

A dyspraxia
B short-term impairment of perceptual motor skills
C paraesthesiae
D short-term memory loss
E headache.

2.31 Important contributions to the study of infantile autism have been made by

A Kanner
B Hermelin
C Connolly
D Goodyer
E Rutter.

2.32 The following names are associated with the development of convulsive therapy

A Cade
B Meduna
C Eysenck
D Bini
E Cerletti.

2.33 Concerning homicide in the UK

A there is a marked association with epilepsy
B approximately one-quarter of victims are aged under 16
C homicide by men is commoner than by women
D there is a marked association with alcohol
E victims have usually been known to the offender.

2.34 The following are matters of civil law in which psychiatrists have special responsibility and can be asked to submit a psychiatric written report

A testamentary capacity
B torts and contracts
C offences against the state
D fitness to drive
E guardianship.

2.35 With respect to paedophiles

A the vast majority of offenders are male
B the victims are not usually known to the offender
C there are approximately equal numbers of male and female victims
D the reconviction rate is high
E older offenders are generally less likely to be aggressive.

2.36   The following are associated with Sigmund Freud
A   repression as the core of symptom formation
B   anima
C   masculine protest
D   free association
E   persona.

2.37   According to Karen Horney, auxiliary methods to relieve inner tension include
A   alienation from self
B   expansiveness
C   self-effacement
D   externalization
E   psychic fragmentation.

2.38   Concepts associated with Alfred Adler include
A   archetypes
B   syntaxic mode
C   organ inferiority
D   locomotor–genital stage
E   masculine protest.

2.39   The following are correctly paired
A   Sullivan: client-centred psychotherapy
B   Klein: play analysis
C   Jung: School of Analytical Psychology
D   Rank: bioenergetics
E   Janov: primal energy.

2.40   Features of homocystinuria include
A   dissecting aortic aneurysm
B   malar flush
C   kyphoscoliosis
D   increased plasma cystine level
E   increased plasma methionine level.

2.41   Down's syndrome
A   is more common in females
B   occurs in 1 in 600 live births
C   usually has severe mental retardation as a feature
D   is associated with an increased incidence of duodenal obstruction
E   is associated with Brushfield spots.

2.42   Recognized viral causes of mental retardation include

   A   rubella
   B   cytomegalovirus
   C   syphilis
   D   toxoplasmosis
   E   yaws.

2.43   Anorexia nervosa

   A   is associated with shoplifting
   B   is associated with depressive symptoms
   C   has a later peak onset in males than in females
   D   never causes death
   E   is associated with a lowered level of luteinizing hormone.

2.44   Features of delirium tremens include

   A   insomnia
   B   leucocytosis
   C   hyperkalaemia
   D   constricted pupils
   E   visual hallucinations.

2.45   Class A drugs under the Misuse of Drugs Act (1971) include

   A   LSD
   B   morphine
   C   cocaine
   D   a preparation of amphetamines for intravenous injection
   E   a preparation of amphetamines for oral use.

2.46   Characteristic features of solvent abuse include the following

   A   more common in males
   B   solitary abuse is common in teenagers
   C   blurred vision occurs during intoxication
   D   tricyclic antidepressants are an effective treatment
   E   hallucinations are usually auditory.

2.47   Recognized features of autoerotic asphyxiation include

   A   more common in females
   B   masturbating while hanging
   C   associated with affective disorders
   D   associated with schizophrenia
   E   associated with transvestism.

2.48   Recognized symptoms of the premenstrual syndrome include

   A   depression
   B   anxiety
   C   fatigue
   D   craving for sweets
   E   constipation.

2.49 Recognized features of systematic desensitization include
  A inflicting pain in the presence of a stimulus
  B phobic hierarchy
  C sleep deprivation
  D flooding
  E relaxation.

2.50 Modelling is a recognized method for
  A treating insomnia
  B treating obsessive–compulsive disorders
  C treating phobic disorders
  D increasing self-assertiveness
  E developing social skills.

PAPER 3: SHORT-ANSWER QUESTION PAPER

3.1 List five organic causes of each of the following:
  a. depression;
  b. episodes of disturbed behaviour.

3.2 a. By whom was bulimia nervosa described?
  b. Name two principal components of this condition.
  c. Name two differential diagnoses.

3.3 Define functional nocturnal enuresis.
  What measures can be taken to help in the management of a
  case of enuresis?

3.4 Write short notes on five important aspects of homocystinuria.

3.5 List factors considered curative in group psychotherapy
  (Yalom).

3.6 List and briefly describe five culture-bound syndromes.

3.7 List five causes of and three clinical features commonly present
  in Korsakoff's psychosis.

3.8 Define dementia and discuss briefly the clinical features of
  senile dementia of the Alzheimer type.

3.9 What factors may influence the response of a patient to a
  physical illness? Outline the various patterns of response which
  may be seen.

3.10 List factors that predict the repetition of deliberate self-
  poisoning.

3.11 What is the difference between validity and reliability as applied to research and statistical methodology?
List three types of each.

3.12 Discuss briefly the disadvantages of making diagnoses in psychiatry.

3.13 State briefly what is meant by the terms autosomal dominant, autosomal recessive and sex-linked inheritance.
For each of these modes of inheritance, name two examples of diseases which may cause mental disorder.

3.14 Name the stages in the biosynthesis of noradrenaline from L-tyrosine.
For each stage, name one inhibitor.

3.15 List the hormones produced by the anterior and posterior lobes of the pituitary gland. For the latter, state the nucleus mainly responsible for the neurosecretion of each hormone.

3.16 Outline briefly the innervation of the extrinsic muscles of the eye by cranial nerves. State briefly what effect occurs on the functioning of the eye when each of these cranial nerves is damaged.

3.17 Give three advantages of the use of benzodiazepines as anxiolytics instead of barbiturates.
List seven side-effects of orally administered benzodiazepines.

3.18 Discuss briefly the stage in cognitive development described by Piaget, giving the approximate ages for each stage.

3.19 List the features which comprise the neuroleptic malignant syndrome.
Name one characteristic serum enzyme change.

3.20 Define the term intelligence quotient.
Name two scales that can be used to measure the intelligence quotient, and, for one the them, list five of the items measured.

PAPER 4: MULTIPLE CHOICE QUESTIONS ON BASIC SCIENCES

4.1 **Piaget descibed the following stages in cognitive development**
  A   latency stage
  B   sensorimotor stage
  C   phallic stage
  D   Electra stage
  E   concrete operational stage.

SWANSEA PSYCHIATRIC EDUCATION LIBRARY

4.2   Gender identity is

A   surgically reversible
B   morphological sex
C   the child's belief as to what sex he or she is
D   partly dependent on parental attitudes
E   sex-typed behaviour patterns.

4.3   The following are part of classical psychoanalytic phases of psychosexual development

A   Electra complex
B   sensorimotor phase
C   anal phase
D   homosexual phase
E   individuation phase.

4.4   Types of activity that may represent displacement activity in certain situations include

A   inappropriate eating
B   doodling
C   sleeping
D   sucking one's thumb
E   fidgeting.

4.5   In connection with systematic desensitization

A   a strict hierarchical presentation is essential
B   the patient should be trained to relax
C   it is a form of reciprocal inhibition
D   phobic disorders are an indication
E   it is a form of aversion therapy.

4.6   Imprinting

A   occurs soon after birth
B   affects adult mating behaviour
C   is seen in the young of nidifugous birds
D   is a mechanism whereby a chick recognizes its mother
E   was first described by Bowlby.

4.7   Features of dysfunction of the parietal lobe include

A   contralateral homonymous hemianopia
B   dressing apraxia
C   dyscalculia
D   sensory dysphasia
E   hypersomnia.

4.8   REM sleep is increased by

A   diazepam
B   electroconvulsive therapy
C   nortriptyline
D   lithium carbonate
E   amphetamines.

4.9   The following substances lead to dilatation of the pupils

A β_1-receptor agonists
B β_2-receptor agonists
C   diamorphine
D   atropine
E   adrenaline.

4.10   The following are intermediates in the biosynthesis of noradrenaline

A   phenylalanine
B   dopamine
C   adrenalin
D   tryptophan
E   acetylcholine.

4.11   Slow activity on the EEG is caused by

A   delirious states
B   nortriptyline
C   lorazepam
D   dementia
E   chloral hydrate.

4.12   Hormones produced by the posterior pituitary include

A   prolactin
B   antidiurectic hormone
C   somatotrophin
D   vasopressin
E   oxytocin.

4.13   The following are neurotransmitters in the central nervous system

A   GABA
B   acetylcholine
C   melatonin
D   bombesin
E   vasoactive intestinal polypeptide.

4.14 Functions of the limbic system include
- A sleep induction
- B awakening
- C sexual activity
- D memory
- E aggressive behaviour.

4.15 5-HT is
- A produced from L-tryptophan
- B found in blood platelets
- C mainly found in the brain
- D metabolized to 5-HIAA
- E metabolized by monoamine oxidase.

4.16 Noradrenaline
- A is produced from tryptophan
- B has a major site in the pons
- C is metabolized to homovanillic acid
- D is metabolized by COMT
- E is released in a calcium-dependent process.

4.17 Acetylcholine is a transmitter at
- A sympathetic ganglia
- B parasympathetic ganglia
- C the adrenal medulla
- D postganglionic sympathetic neuroeffector junctions
- E bronchodilator sympathetic nerves.

4.18 The following are intermediates in the biosynthesis of histamine
- A tryptophan
- B imidozole acetic acid
- C hydroxytryptamine
- D histidine
- E hydroxyhistamine.

4.19 Catechol-O-methyltransferase is involved in the metabolism of
- A serotonin
- B dopamine
- C noradrenaline
- D acetylcholine
- E lithium.

4.20 Opioid sigma receptors are probably involved in
- A miosis
- B sedation
- C respiratory depression
- D dysphoria
- E hallucinations.

4.21 Side-effects of neuroleptics include

A   akathisia
B   oculogyric crisis
C   shortened ventricular repolarization on the ECG
D   torticollis
E   diarrhoea.

4.22 Haloperidol differs from chlorpromazine in that

A   it has no antiemetic effect
B   it has no anticholinergic effect
C   it has a greater-tendency to cause hypotension
D   it is less likely to cause urinary retention
E   it is less likely to cause dystonic reactions.

4.23 Side-effects of diazepam include

A   dry mouth
B   headache
C   respiratory stimulation
D   ataxia
E   insomnia.

4.24 L-tryptophan

A   is an antidepressant
B   should never be given with monoamine oxidase inhibitors
C   induces hepatic tryptophan pyrolase
D   is a 5-HT precursor
E   is an amino acid.

4.25 Foods to avoid while being treated with monomine oxidase inhibitors include

A   pickled herring
B   cottage cheese
C   yeast extract
D   game
E   wines.

4.26 The prevalence of the following is higher in members of social class V than social class I

A   anorexia nervosa
B   antisocial behaviour
C   parasuicide
D   male suicides over the age of 65
E   cerebrovascular disease.

4.27   Experimental studies tend to indicate that, compared with middle-class subjects, lower-class subjects show less

A   control over impluses
B   likelihood to blame others for their failures
C   ability to persevere at difficult tasks
D   ability to postpone gratifications
E   self-interest.

4.28   Total institutions is a term which

A   was used following a study of St Elizabeth's Hospital, Washington, DC
B   was used by Goffman
C   includes prisons
D   includes day schools
E   includes convents.

4.29   The International Pilot Study of Schizophrenia showed that

A   outcome was more favourable in developing countries than in developed ones
B   schizophrenia has a higher prevalence in developing countries than in developed ones
C   American psychiatrists had an unusually broad concept of schizophrenia
D   Russian psychiatrists has an unusually broad concept of schizophernia
E   Danish, Nigerian, Indian and British psychiatrists showed a similar concept of schizophernia.

4.30   Sick-role behaviour includes the following types of behaviour

A   undergoing a health check-up
B   looking for a suitable remedy
C   attempting to define the state of one's health
D   attempting to prevent disease
E   activity adopted when one considers oneself to be ill.

4.31   In Belknap's sociological study of an American psychiatric hospital in the the 1950s, patients were found to fall into the following categories

A   apathetic
B   compliant
C   overcompliant
D   co-operative
E   troublesome.

4.32   A Barr body is seen in nuclei of cells from the following

A   normal male
B   normal female
C   Turner's syndrome
D   Klinefelter's syndrome
E   XYY syndrome.

4.33   The following are recessive conditions

A   galactosaemia
B   amaurotic idiocy
C   tuberous sclerosis
D   homocystinuria
E   phenylketonuria.

4.34   In cell division

A   the number of chromosomes in germ cells in haploid
B   the number of chromosomes in a zygote is aneuploid
C   germ cell double cell division is called mitosis
D   human gametes are diploid
E   the normal human female karyotype is 44XX.

4.35   A sex chromosome abnormality demonstrable by microscopic techniques is characteristically associated with

A   Klinefelter's syndrome
B   Turner's syndrome
C   Patau's syndrome
D   Niemann–Pick disease
E   Lesch–Nyhan syndrome.

4.36   Dizygotic twins

A   characteristically share a greater proportion of their genes than full siblings
B   arise from two separate ova
C   have a higher concordance rate than monozygotic twins for speaking Japanese in Tokyo
D   have a higher concordance rate than monozygotic twins for schizophrenia
E   have the same concordance rate as monozygotic twins for alcoholism.

4.37   The XYY syndrome is associated with

A   lower intelligence
B   lower height
C   being imprisoned more often
D   being chromatin-negative
E   an incidence of approximately 1 in 700 births.

4.38 Phenylketonuria is associated with

A blue eyes
B microcephaly
C elevated plasma phenylalanine
D an abnormal EEG
E a deficiency of phenylalanine hydroxylase.

4.39 According to T. Szasz

A illness is defined by the presence of suffering
B most mental disorders are illnesses
C most mental disorders are the province of doctors
D those who are suicidal should have the right to refuse treatment
E a role behaviour model is more appropriate than the medical model in explaining some hysterical disorders.

4.40 Psychoses

A include general paralysis of the insane
B include delirium tremens
C include obsessive–compulsive disorders
D feature symptoms including hallucinations
E feature symptoms including lack of insight.

4.41 DSM-III R

A has five axes
B axes I and II are not categorical
C axis II includes personality disorders
D axis IV rates psychological stress
E has more detailed definitions than ICD 9.

4.42 Suicide rates

A are highest during April to June in England and Wales
B are highest during April to June in Australia
C increase with increasing age
D are higher in men than women at all ages
E are highest in social classes I and V compared with the other social classes.

4.43 Occupations in which there is an increased risk of alcohol dependence include

A kitchen porters
B brewery workers
C executives
D seamen
E entertainers.

4.44   The classification of the neuroses in ICD 9 includes

A   conversion disorder
B   psychogenic disorder
C   panic disorder
D   agoraphobia
E   dysthymic disorder.

4.45   In a frequency curve

A   height represents the frequency of a class interval
B   the dependent variable increases as the independent variable increases
C   data are represented as a histogram
D   frequency corresponds to a width of class interval
E   total frequency equals the maximum height.

4.46   A test is carried out and the mean score is 100 and the standard deviation is 20 in the population, and the scores are normally distributed. The following are true

A   the median score is 100
B   approximately 95% of scores are in the range 60–140
C   the probability of scoring more than 100 is 0.75
D   the probability of scoring between 94 and 106 inclusive is approximately 0.5
E   the mode is greater than 100.

4.47   The following are measures of variation

A   variance
B   null hypothesis
C   mode
D   standard deviation
E   range.

4.48   Patients are randomly allocated to two groups. One of these groups is then chosen at random and its members are given a trial drug. Differences later found between the two groups are probably not caused by

A   instrumentation
B   selection
C   the trial drug
D   maturation–selection interaction
E   history.

4.49   Tests that assume a normal distribution of the measured variable in the population include

A   Mann–Whitney U test
B   analysis of variance
C   Student's t-test
D   Wilcoxon's rank sum test
E   chi-squared test.

4.50   The standard deviation is

    A the difference between the largest and smallest observations in a sample

    B a good measure of variability or spread when the distribution is Gaussian

    C a good measure of variability or spread when the distribution is skewed to the right

    D not a good measure of variability or spread when the distribution is both symmetrical and bimodal

    E the variance squared.

PAPER 5: MULTIPLE CHOICE QUESTIONS ON CLINICAL TOPICS

5.1   Delirious patients

    A are rarely disorientated for time

    B experience illusions

    C are best nursed in very brightly lit rooms

    D may show overactivity

    E have unimpaired insight.

5.2   Concerning Huntington's chorea

    A it is commoner in women

    B it causes basal ganglia atrophy

    C epilepsy occurs especially in older patients

    D insight is impaired early in the course of the disease

    E depression is common.

5.3   Following head injury

    A the period of retrograde amnesia is a good predictor of outcome

    B the rate of development of a schizophrenia-like syndrome is increased

    C there is no increase in the risk of suicide

    D personality change may occur

    E the duration of post-traumatic amnesia is related to the degree of psychiatric disability.

5.4   The following drugs may be given to a patient who has acute intermittent porphyria

    A diazepam

    B barbiturates

    C digoxin

    D chlorpromazine

    E griseofulvin.

5.5   Intracerebral calcification is associated with the following conditions

A   hypoparathyroidism
B   pseudohypoparathyroidism
C   glioblastoma multiforme
D   angioma
E   tuberous sclerosis.

5.6   Recognized features of aspirin overdose include

A   hyperventilation
B   vasodilatation
C   tinnitus
D   sweating
E   deafness.

5.7   Recognized causes of parkinsonism include

A   manganese poisoning
B   the 'punch-drunk' syndrome
C   sphenoidal ridge meningiomas
D   meningovascular syphilis
E   encephalitis lethargica.

5.8   Pica

A   gets worse with age
B   includes geophagia
C   is usually treated with neuroleptic medication
D   is associated with emotional distress
E   is associated with brain damage.

5.9   With regard to hysteria in children

A   it is less common in adolescence than in younger children as an individual illness
B   it is less common in adolescence than in younger children in its epidemic form
C   childhood symptoms are usually mild
D   symptoms include paralysis
E   symptoms include abnormality of gait.

5.10   Compared with school refusers, Hersov found that truants

A   came from more neurotic families
B   were more passive
C   were more depressed
D   were more overprotected
E   had better records of school work.

5.11   The term hyperkinetic syndrome, as used in Britain, includes the following features

A   it is less common in girls
B   it is associated with epilepsy
C   it is associated with intellectual retardation
D   treatment with benzodiazepines is often effective
E   it never persists from childhood into adult life.

5.12   Children with infantile autism

A   do better with a structured education
B   are more likely to have schizophrenic parents
C   have normal cognitive function
D   become less withdrawn with age
E   are likely to develop epilepsy in adolescence.

5.13   Dimensions used in Sjobring's classification include

A   reliability
B   stability
C   capacity
D   validity
E   solidity.

5.14   Recognized features of overbreathing during an anxiety attack include

A   headache
B   paraesthesiae
C   carpopedal spasm
D   dizziness
E   precordial discomfort.

5.15   As compared with agoraphobia, in social phobic neurosis

A   depression occurs more often
B   obsessions occur more often
C   depersonalization occurs more often
D   alcohol abuse is commoner
E   patients rarely feel anxious in advance of encountering anxiety-causing situations.

5.16   Characteristic dissociative hysterical symptoms include

A   paralysis
B   amnesia
C   convulsions
D   fugue
E   multiple personality.

5.17   **Conditions that can present with depression include**
   A   hyperparathyroidism
   B   Addison's disease
   C   Cushing's disease
   D   acromegaly
   E   hypothyroidism.

5.18   **Recognized symptoms of mania include**
   A   schneiderian first-rank symptoms
   B   delusions of reference
   C   passivity feelings
   D   auditory hallucinations
   E   Cotard's syndrome.

5.19   **Factors predicting a poor prognosis in schizophrenia include**
   A   no past psychiatric history
   B   blunted affect
   C   social isolation
   D   sudden onset
   E   being widowed.

5.20   **Changes that occur in the brain with ageing include**
   A   decrease in weight
   B   decrease in ventricular size
   C   decrease in meningeal thickness
   D   increase in senile plaques
   E   a major loss of nerve cells.

5.21   **The Gresham Ward Questionnaire**
   A   assesses memory for general events
   B   assesses memory for recent personal events
   C   gives an indication of the severity of intellectual handicap
   D   is used with psychogeriatric patients
   E   assesses memory for past personal events.

5.22   **Clinical features of the early stages of senile dementia of the Alzheimer type include**
   A   loss of spincter control
   B   minor forgetfulness
   C   disorientation
   D   waking at night
   E   paranoid delusions.

5.23   **The Ganser syndrome**
   A   was described in 1898
   B   is characterized by the phenomenon of *vorbeigehen*
   C   is characterized by hallucinations
   D   is characterized by apparent clouding of consciousness
   E   was first described among prisoners.

5.24   Factors that are related to how effective lithium will be as a prophylactic in affective disorders include

A   sex
B   age of onset of the first episode of affective disorder
C   a family history of affective disorder
D   age at start of lithium therapy
E   number of previous episodes of affective disorder.

5.25   In the 6 months following a life event, Paykel found that

A   the relative risk for schizophrenia is approximately 7
B   the risk for depression is greater than the risk for schizophrenia
C   the risk for neurosis is greater than the risk for attempted suicide
D   the risk for suicide attempts is greater than the risk for schizophrenia
E   the relative risk is a poor measure of the magnitude of the causative effect of life event stress.

5.26   The following statements concerning the epidemiology of mental retardation in Britain are true

A   in the population aged 15–19, the prevalence of moderate and severe retardation is greater than 3 per 1000
B   the prevalence of moderate and severe retardation fell by approximately one-third between the 1930s and the 1960s
C   the incidence of severe retardation changed little between the 1930s and the 1960s
D   the administrative prevalence increases after the age of 16
E   the relative frequencies of psychiatric symptoms and syndromes are significantly greater among those with mild mental retardation than in people of normal intelligence.

5.27   Contraindications to therapy with beta-adrenoreceptor antagonists include

A   intermittent claudication
B   metabolic acidosis
C   prolonged fasting as in anorexia nervosa
D   a history of asthma
E   heart block.

5.28   Side effects of tricyclic antidepressant drugs include

A   fine tremor
B   peripheral neuropathy
C   inco-ordination
D   depressed ST segments on the ECG
E   shortened QT interval on the ECG.

5.29 Contraindications to ECT include
A   pregnancy
B   cerebral oedema
C   age under 12
D   old age
E   raised intracranial pressure.

5.30 The following names are associated with theories of thought disorder
A   Goldstein
B   Payne
C   Friedlander
D   Fregoli
E   Cameron.

5.31 The following names are associated with the development of psychosurgical techniques
A   Lima
B   Lewis
C   Watts
D   Moniz
E   Ferenczi.

5.32 Important contributions to the study of sleep disorders have been made by
A   Gardner
B   Yalom
C   Roth
D   Zarcone
E   Oswald.

5.33 Homicide is 'normal' if the legal outcome is
A   infanticide
B   common law manslaughter
C   suicide murder
D   diminished responsibility
E   murder.

5.34 Crimes closely associated with mental retardation include
A   blackmail
B   homicide
C   arson
D   theft
E   indecent exposure.

5.35   Conditions associated with shoplifting include

A   depression
B   mania
C   anorexia nervosa
D   acute schizophrenia
E   phobic anxiety.

5.36   Concepts associated with Erik Erikson include the following

A   reality principle
B   animus
C   identity crisis
D   self-esteem
E   epigenesis.

5.37   Carl Jung wrote

A   Persuasion and healing
B   The interpretation of dreams
C   The ego and the id
D   The theory and practice of group psychotherapy
E   The basic fault.

5.38   The psychodynamic theory of the trauma of birth

A   is a concept developed by Otto Rank
B   refers to the maternal pain of labour
C   is the same as individuation
D   gives rise to primal anxiety
E   is a central archetype.

5.39   Therapeutic factors in supportive group psychotherapy include

A   instruction
B   caring attitude
C   permission for display of emotion
D   environmental manipulation
E   scapegoating.

5.40   Factors involved in psychoanalytic cure identified by M. Gitelson include

A   insight
B   recall of infantile memories
C   hypnosis
D   catharsis
E   the relationship with the analyst.

5.41   Recognized perinatal causes of mental retardation include

A   kernicterus
B   intraventricular haemorrhage
C   exposure to radiation
D   toxoplasmosis
E   lead intoxication.

5.42   Recognized features of the fetal alcohol syndrome include

   A   postnatal growth deficiency
   B   microcephaly
   C   mental retardation
   D   shortened palpebral fissure
   E   maxillary hypoplasia.

5.43   Bulimia nervosa

   A   was first described by William Gull
   B   never occurs in males
   C   has bereavement as a recognized precipitating factor
   D   has first sexual intercourse as a recognized precipitating factor
   E   never occurs in non-whites.

5.44   Schedule 1 of the Misuse of Drugs Regulations (1985) includes the following drugs

   A   heroin
   B   barbiturates
   C   cannabis
   D   pentazocine
   E   lysergide.

5.45   Under the Misuse of Drugs (Notification of and Supply to Addicts) Regulations (1973) a medical practitioner must notify the Chief Medical Officer (London or Belfast) of any person believed to be addicted to

   A   cannabis
   B   cocaine
   C   pethidine
   D   LSD
   E   methadone.

5.46   Diseases that cause erectile impotence include

   A   acromegaly
   B   mumps
   C   diabetes mellitus
   D   plumbism
   E   Klinefelter's syndrome.

5.47   Exhibitionists characteristically

   A   rape their victims
   B   practise voyeurism
   C   choose places where they risk detection
   D   respond to electrical aversion therapy
   E   respond to group psychotherapy.

5.48   Recognized forms of behaviour therapy include
    A   response prevention
    B   modelling
    C   implosive therapy
    D   imprinting
    E   habit reversal.

5.49   Types of aversion therapy include
    A   classical conditioning
    B   biofeedback
    C   covert sensitization
    D   overcorrection
    E   escape and avoidance learning.

5.50   Biofeedback techniques can enable control to be gained over the following
    A   EEG activity
    B   single motor unit firing
    C   blood pressure
    D   pulse amplitude
    E   skin temperature.

PAPER 6: SHORT-ANSWER QUESTION PAPER

6.1   Discuss briefly the stages seen in typical uncomplicated bereavement.
List three ways in which the features seen in uncomplicated bereavement differ from those seen in depressive disorders.

6.2   List Schneider's first-rank symptoms of schizophrenia. Comment briefly on their prognostic value.

6.3   Write short notes on five major features of school refusal in children.

6.4   List the criteria that should be used to determine the testamentary capacity of a person suffering from mental disorder.

6.5   List 10 ego defence mechanisms.

6.6   What is delirium tremens?
List seven clinical features commonly present in this condition, and state one electrolyte disturbance that commonly occurs.

6.7   Discuss briefly the treatment of manic-depressive psychoses in the elderly.

6.8   List five organic causes of each of the following:
a. anxiety;
b. fatigue.

6.9   Briefly outline the features of the treatment technique for sexual dysfunction introduced by Masters and Johnson.

6.10   Describe briefly, under five headings, some important features of complex partial seizures.

6.11   Define the following terms used in statistical tests:
a. null hypothesis;
b. type 1 error;
c. type 2 error;
d. power.

6.12   a. Briefly outline two genetic mechanisms that may cause Down's syndrome.
b. List eight clinical features common in this condition.

6.13   What is the dopamine hypothesis of schizophrenia?
Briefly list evidence that supports this hypothesis.

6.14   List the principal components of the limbic system and state three of its normal functions.

6.15   What is meant by the term dysarthria?
List six possible causes.

6.16   Discuss briefly Eysenck's theory of personality.

6.17   Under each of the following headings, list five side-effects of lithium carbonate:
a. early;
b. toxicity;
c. long-term.

6.18   Describe briefly procedures that can be employed to avoid bias in the outcome of a clinical trial.

6.19   a. Name two neuronal groups thought to be involved in causing sleep.
b. List characteristics of REM sleep.

6.20   Discuss briefly Sigmund Freud's stages of psychosexual development, giving the approximate ages for each stage.

PAPER 7: MULTIPLE CHOICE QUESTIONS ON BASIC SCIENCES

7.1   An average 8-month-old child

A   shows social smiling
B   is beginning to enter the oedipal complex
C   speaks in phrases
D   is beginning to show stranger anxiety
E   is beginning to show separation anxiety.

7.2   The following are terms used in ethology

A   species-specific behaviour
B   imprinting
C   cognitive dissonance
D   Gestalt
E   late-maturing complex behaviour.

7.3   Common precipitants of aggression include

A   low social class
B   poverty
C   pain
D   fustration
E   having hostile repressive parents.

7.4   The development of language in humans

A   is often impaired in institutionalized children
B   passes through the babbling stage which occurs also in the congenitally deaf
C   reaches basic adult grammar by age 36 months
D   reaches 2–3 word sentences by age 12 months
E   is related to measured intelligence.

7.5   Cognitive dissonance

A   was described by Bannister
B   arises when two cognitions occurring together are inconsistent with each other
C   resolution leads to decreased internal discomfort
D   is usually recognized by the subject
E   may be reduced by adding new cognitions which are consonant with pre-existing ones.

7.6   Personality tests include

A   WISC
B   Cattell 16PF
C   MMPI
D   WAIS
E   thematic apperception test.

7.7   Features of dysfunction of the temporal lobe include
- A   schizophrenia-like psychosis
- B   topographical agnosia
- C   emotional lability
- D   contralateral spastic paresis
- E   upper quadrant contralateral homonymous hemianopia.

7.8   Gerstmann's syndrome
- A   includes dressing apraxia
- B   includes finger agnosia
- C   occurs in dominant temporal lobe lesions
- D   includes disinhibition
- E   includes dysgraphia.

7.9   The transmitter at
- A   parasympathetic postganglionic nerve endings is muscarine
- B   parasympathetic ganglia is sometimes noradrenaline
- C   sympathetic ganglia is nicotine
- D   sympathetic postganglionic nerve endings is always noradrenaline
- E   the parasympathetic innervation of the adrenal medulla is acetylcholine.

7.10   The following are intermediates in the biosynthesis of dopamine
- A   tryptophan
- B   dihydroxyphenylalanine
- C   phenylalanine
- D   homovanillic acid
- E   dihydroxyglycolic aldehyde.

7.11   The following substances may be excitatory central neurotransmitters
- A   vasoactive intestinal peptide
- B   histamine
- C   gamma-aminobutyric acid
- D   glutamic acid
- E   somatostatin.

7.12   The following nuclei are associated with neurosecretion
- A   caudate
- B   supraoptic
- C   lenticular
- D   amygdala
- E   paraventricular.

7.13   The limbic system includes

    A   dentate gyrus
    B   cerebellum
    C   hypothalamus
    D   amygdaloid nucleus
    E   subcallosal gyrus.

7.14   Constriction of the pupils in response to light involves the following structures

    A   cerebral cortex
    B   optic tracts
    C   ciliary ganglia
    D   lateral geniculate nuclei
    E   Edinger–Westphal nuclei.

7.15   The following structures lie within the metencephalon

    A   pons
    B   pituitary gland
    C   crura cerebri
    D   cerebellum
    E   basal ganglia.

7.16   The following are neurotransmitter breakdown products

    A   hydroxyindolacetic acid
    B   homovanillic acid
    C   imidazole acetic acid
    D   3-methoxy-4-hydroxyphenylglycol
    E   dopamine.

7.17   Monoamine oxidase is involved in the metabolism of

    A   noradrenaline
    B   dopamine
    C   acetylcholine
    D   5-hydroxytryptamine
    E   glutamic acid.

7.18   Opioid μ-receptors are probably involved in

    A   physical dependence on opioids
    B   spinal analgesia
    C   euphoria
    D   hallucinations
    E   respiratory depression.

7.19   Chlorpromazine

    A   antagonizes the action of dopamine
    B   antagonizes the action of noradrenaline
    C   decreases the level of prolactin
    D   is strongly anticholinergic
    E   is an α-adrenoreceptor antagonist.

7.20   Side-effects of neuroleptic medication include
A   dry mouth
B   hypertensive crisis
C   menstrual cycle disturbances
D   blurred vision
E   opisthotonus.

7.21   Abrupt withdrawal of benzodiazepines used in high dosage may lead to
A   emotional disorders
B   confusion
C   epileptiform seizures
D   toxic psychosis
E   a condition resembling delirium tremens.

7.22   Cannabis
A   causes physical dependence
B   causes psychic dependence
C   causes formication
D   has as its active substance trihydro-cannabinol
E   causes euphoria.

7.23   Side-effects of tricyclic antidepressants include
A   bradycardia
B   hypertensive crisis
C   paralytic ileus
D   jaundice
E   diarrhoea.

7.24   Side-effects of monoamine oxidase inhibitors include
A   psychotic episodes
B   increased REM sleep
C   epilepsy
D   failure of ejaculation
E   blurred vision.

7.25   Social class II includes the following occupations
A   radiographers
B   lawyers
C   social workers
D   landowners
E   nurses.

7.26 A therapeutic community
  A   is a term first used by Maxwell Jones
  B   involves the absence of rigid hierarchies
  C   is provided at the Henderson Hospital
  D   was a term first used to describe the regime at the Cassel Hospital
  E   shows that patients are unable to play a useful role in their treatment.

7.27 The following are culture-bound syndromes
  A   schizophrenia
  B   amok
  C   latah
  D   windigo
  E   koro.

7.28 Institutional neurosis
  A   was a term first used by Barton
  B   includes withdrawal of interest
  C   refers to the clinical effects of poor hospital care
  D   is treatable
  E   may increase in severity with duration of stay in hospital.

7.29 The following are forms of marriage
  A   polyandry
  B   exogamy
  C   polygyny
  D   endogamy
  E   polygamy.

7.30 Vulnerability factors identified by Brown & Harris (1978) following their studies of depressed women in London include
  A   maternal loss before the age of 11
  B   young children at home
  C   lack of a confiding relationship with a husband or partner
  D   no job outside the home
  E   being working class.

7.31 Individuals with Klinefelter' syndrome
  A   have one Y chromosome in the genetic constitution
  B   have one X chromosome in the genetic constitution
  C   are chromatin-negative
  D   tend to be withdrawn and timid
  E   are often sterile.

7.32   The following are recessive conditions

A   maple syrup urine disease
B   histidinaemia
C   Hartnup's disease
D   von Recklinghausen's disease
E   Niemann–Pick disease.

7.33   The following may show autosomal dominant transmission

A   familial fructose intolerance
B   Hurler's syndrome
C   Wilson's disease
D   epiloia
E   Sturge–Weber syndrome.

7.34   The following conditions are characteristically associated with autosomal chromosomal trisomy

A   cri du chat
B   Down's syndrome
C   Patau's syndrome
D   Hunter's syndrome
E   'Edward's syndrome.

7.35   Polygenic inheritance

A   is a mendelian pattern of inheritance
B   is mediated by the additive action of a number of genes, each of small effect
C   is entirely responsible for human stature
D   with a threshold, gives a model with which spina bifida fits
E   may occur in schizophrenia.

7.36   The following are disorders of the urea cycle which are associated with mental retardation

A   homocystinuria
B   citrullinuria
C   hyperammonaemia
D   argininosuccinicaciduria
E   Hartnup's disease.

7.37   Turner's syndrome

A   may coexist with Duchenne muscular dystrophy
B   is usually associated with absent pubic hair
C   may be caused by sex chromosomal non-dysjunction
D   patients never have menstrual bleeding
E   is associated with coarctation of the aorta.

7.38   For the purposes of legal requirements, most psychiatrists would not include the following categories in the concept of mental illness

A   homosexuality
B   personality disorder
C   drug abuse
D   fetishism
E   mental handicap.

7.39   The following populations have a high prevalence of schizophrenia

A   inhabitants of the extreme north of Sweden
B   inhabitants of north-west Yugoslavia
C   American Hutterites
D   Canadian Roman Catholics
E   South Indian Tamils.

7.40   The classification of neurosis in ICD 9 includes

A   phobic states
B   somatoform disorders
C   dissociative disorders
D   factitious disorders
E   neurotic depression.

7.41   Suicide rates are higher in

A   widowers than in the divorced
B   the married than in the never-married
C   widows than in widowers
D   the divorced than in the never-married
E   the unemployed than in the employed.

7.42   Occupations in which there is an increased risk of alcohol-related disability include

A   doctors
B   publicans
C   chefs
D   actors
E   printers.

7.43   The following are features of the normal distribution

A   the median occasionally coincides with the mode
B   it is symmetrical
C   the mean is greater than the mode
D   approximately 95% of the total population lies within one standard deviation of the mean
E   over 99% of the total population lies within two standard deviations of the mean.

7.44 Parametric statistical tests include

    A Spearman rank-order correlation
    B sign test
    C Mann–Whitney U test
    D two-sample t-test
    E Kolmogorov–Smirnov test.

7.45 From a given population, a sample of 16 people is chosen at random. They are found to have a mean IQ of 90, with a standard deviation of 12. The following statements are true of this sample

    A the sum of the IQs of this sample is the product of 90 and 16
    B the 95% confidence interval for the population mean is approximately 78 to 102
    C the standard error of the mean is 3
    D to calculate confidence intervals it would be more appropriate to use the normal distribution than the t distribution
    E the variance is 144.

7.46 In double-blind controlled clinical trials

    A more than one controlled group may be used
    B the subject is unaware of which group he or she belongs to
    C the experimenter making the assessments is unaware of which group the subject belongs to
    D each subject receives a placebo treatment
    E each subject receives the new treatment.

7.47 Sources of variation in clinical trials include

    A placebo effect
    B practice effect
    C natural remission
    D Hawthorne effect
    E natural course of illness fluctuation.

7.48 Aspects of the correlation coefficient include the following

    A a correlation coefficient of -1 implies complete absence of correlation
    B a correlation coefficient of $+1$ implies complete correlation
    C the line of best fit would show a negative gradient on a scatter diagram plotting two series of variables against each other when the correlation coefficient between these two sets of variables is less than $+1$
    D the line of best fit would show a positive gradient on a scatter diagram plotting two series of variables against each other when the correlation coefficient between these two sets of variables is equal to $+1$
    E a correlation coefficient of $+1$ implies causation.

7.49   In connection with the chi-squared test
  A   Yate's correction may be used
  B   it may be used to analyse categorical data
  C   it is only valid if the items analysed are uncorrelated
  D   calculation of the statistic chi-squared involves the determination of the number of degrees of freedom
  E   calculation of the value of p involves the determination of the number of degrees of freedom.

7.50   The t-test may be used in the following cases
  A   the determination of the probability that a certain range around the mean of a sample with known standard deviation includes the population mean
  B   the analysis of qualitative categorical data
  C   the calculation of the statistical significance of the difference between the means of two samples whose standard deviations are known
  D   to determine how significantly the mean of a sample of known standard deviation differs from a postulated population mean
  E   to determine the significance of the difference between the means of two sets of paired observations made on two samples.

PAPER 8: MULTIPLE CHOICE QUESTIONS ON CLINICAL TOPICS

8.1   Among the 'exogenous reactions' proposed by Karl Bonhoeffer were
  A   epileptic excitement
  B   twilight state
  C   delirium
  D   amentia
  E   hallucinosis.

8.2   In Huntington's chorea
  A   pallidectomy has been used as a treatment
  B   persecutory delusions may be present
  C   neuronal loss is most marked in the temporal lobes
  D   suicide is common
  E   onset is never before the age of 18.

8.3   The development of a chronic schizophrenia-like syndrome is a recognized association of
  A   cannabis use
  B   complex partial seizures
  C   the postoperative period
  D   alcohol abuse
  E   encephalitis.

8.4   Post-traumatic amnesia

A   is the time between the head injury and the last clearly
     recalled memory before the injury
B   lasting 1 to 7 days was defined as moderate concussion by
     Russell and Smith
C   lasting more than 7 days was defined as severe concussion
     by Russell and Smith
D   duration is closely correlated with neurological
     complications
E   duration is closely correlated with change of personality
     after head injury.

8.5   Recognized features of paracetamol overdose include

A   acute renal failure
B   shortened prothrombin time
C   hyperventilation, usually within 12 hours
D   hepatic failure, usually within 24 hours
E   coma, usually within 24 hours.

8.6   Recognized features of Addison's disease include

A   depression
B   hypertension
C   fatigue
D   hirsuitism
E   mild cognitive impairment.

8.7   The EEG

A   may exclude the diagnosis of epilepsy
B   may be abnormal in schizophrenia
C   may be abnormal in antisocial personality disorder
D   may be helpful in localizing a space-occupying lesion
E   is sensitive to the blood sugar level.

8.8   The following occur in the 'punch-drunk' syndrome

A   dysarthria
B   amnesic confabulation
C   morbid jealousy
D   pyramidal signs
E   increased drive.

8.9   With regard to separation anxiety in children

A   children typically exhibit 'frozen watchfulness'
B   it is a cause of school refusal
C   children may worry that their parents will become ill
D   it is more common in adolescence than in younger children
E   anxiolytic drugs should generally be avoided.

8.10   Regarding obsessive–compulsive neurosis in childhood
A   it is rare
B   avoiding cracks in the pavement is likely to be a symptom
C   touching lamp posts is likely to be a symptom
D   the child may involve its parents
E   the child may seem to cry for no apparent reason.

8.11   Juvenile delinquency
A   is related to poor housing
B   is related to poor education
C   is also known as conduct disorder
D   is a psychiatric diagnosis carrying a good prognosis
E   genetic factors are important.

8.12   Infantile autism
A   is also known as childhood schizophrenia
B   was first described by Rutter
C   has a prevalence of 0.5–1.0% of children
D   is more frequent in lower social classes
E   can be familial.

8.13   The ICD 9 classification of personality disorders includes the following categories
A   paranoid
B   narcissistic
C   borderline
D   passive aggressive
E   asthenic.

8.14   Types of body build described by Kretschmer include
A   athletic
B   leptosomatic
C   viscerotonic
D   pyknic
E   asthenic.

8.15   Recognized features of an anxiety neurosis include
A   amenorrhoea
B   dry mouth
C   excessive wind
D   penile erection
E   urgency of micturition.

8.16   Characteristic conversion hysterical symptoms include
A   aphonia
B   vomiting
C   depersonalization
D   somnabulism
E   pseudocyesis.

8.17   Recognized symptoms of depression include

A   depersonalization
B   poor memory
C   obsessional symptoms
D   phobias
E   fugue.

8.18   Somniloquy

A   is commoner in females
B   occurs during slow-wave sleep
C   is associated with helminthiasis
D   is associated with toxic states
E   is associated with post-traumatic states.

8.19   The first-rank symptoms of schizophrenia include

A   altered body image
B   lack of insight
C   secondary delusions
D   suspiciousness
E   flatness of affect.

8.20   Factors predicting a good prognosis in schizophrenia include

A   good previous personality
B   short episode
C   good record at work
D   younger age at onset
E   prominent affective symptoms.

8.21   In his study on the natural history of mental disorder in old age, Roth (1955) found that

A   late paraphrenia had a better prognosis than senile psychosis
B   arteriosclerotic psychosis had a better prognosis than acute confusion
C   arteriosclerotic psychosis had a better prognosis than affective psychosis
D   acute confusion had a better prognosis than senile. psychosis
E   organic states were diagnosed more often in Britain than in the United States.

8.22   In elderly patients suffering from an acute organic syndrome

A   impairment of consciousness occasionally occurs
B   an important predisposing factor is defective hearing
C   an important predisposing factor is pre-existing dementia
D   mortality is uncommon
E   small doses of benzodiazepines are an appropriate way of providing symptomatic relief.

8.23   Depressive symptoms are more common
  A   in women
  B   in lower socioeconomic groups
  C   among those who are divorced
  D   among those who are separated
  E   during the menopause.

8.24   Concerning the epidemiology of common causes of presenile dementia
  A   systemic lupus erythematosus has a female to male ratio of approximately 9 to 1 in the second and third decades
  B   Alzheimer's disease is the second most common form of presenile dementia
  C   the prevalence of Huntington's chorea is approximately 4 to 7 per 10 000
  D   men and women are affected in equal numbers by Pick's disease
  E   Alzheimer's disease and Huntington's chorea are more common in women.

8.25   Concerning alcohol consumption in the UK
  A   the lowest point in the per caput consumption of all forms of alcohol since the 17th century was reached after the Second World War
  B   the per caput consumption of alcohol was higher in the 1970s than it was in the late 19th century
  C   drinking amongst women has tended to stay fairly constant in the second half of the 20th century
  D   the alcohol industry tends to recruit men who are already heavy drinkers
  E   in the 1970s and 1980s there was increased drinking and drunkenness amongst adolescents.

8.26   The studies by Rutter et al on 10- and 11-year-olds in the Isle of Wight found that psychiatric disorder was correlated with
  A   organic brain damage
  B   intelligence
  C   physical handicap
  D   reading retardation
  E   all of the above.

8.27   The following are drugs that should either be avoided or used with caution in breastfeeding mothers
  A   chloral hydrate
  B   meprobamate
  C   amitriptyline
  D   nitrazepam
  E   carbamazepine.

8.28 **During ECT, physiological changes that occur include the following**

A   if no atropine premedication is given, transient cardiac arrhythmias may occur in over 50% of patients

B   if no atropine premedication is given, the pulse rises initially to over 100 beats/minute

C   if a muscle relaxant is given, the systolic blood pressure never reaches 200 mmHg

D   cerebral blood flow may more than double

E   increased cerebral arterial vasoconstriction.

8.29 **Depression is a known side-effect of the following drugs**

A   methyldopa

B   frusemide

C   reserpine

D   co-trimoxazole

E   clonidine.

8.30 **The following names are associated with important contributions to the study of eating disorders**

A   Russell

B   Crisp

C   Morgan

D   Fairburn

E   Lacey.

8.31 **The following names are associated with important studies in the field of psychogeriatrics**

A   Adler

B   Roth

C   Post

D   Blessed

E   Levy.

8.32 **The following are associated**

A   Cade — lithium

B   Deniker — chlorpromazine

C   Kuhn — haloperidol

D   Laborit — chlorpromazine

E   Janssen — chlordiazepoxide.

8.33 **Compared with homicide offenders in general, in acts of homicide followed by suicide in England and Wales the offender is more likely to**

A   be male

B   be of higher social class

C   have had more previous convictions

D   be severely depressed

E   have killed a child or children.

8.34   Fitness to plead

A   can be decided in a magistrates' court
B   can be decided by a jury
C   includes the ability to understand the proceedings in court
D   includes the ability to instruct counsel for the defence
E   includes the ability to understand the nature of the charge.

8.35   Sigmund Freud wrote the following works

A   Memories, dreams, reflections
B   Symbols of transformation
C   Introductory lectures on psychoanalysis
D   The interpretation of dreams
E   The ego and the mechanisms of defence.

8.36   The following concepts were developed by Harry Stack Sullivan

A   self-system
B   parataxic distortion
C   depressive position
D   prototaxic thinking
E   gestalt.

8.37   Complexes described by Jung include

A   inferiority complex
B   shadow
C   collective unconscious
C   animus
E   persona.

8.38   Melanie Klein is associated with the development of the following concepts

A   depressive position
B   idealization
C   projective identification
D   paranoid–schizoid position
E   splitting.

8.39   Wilhelm Reich is associated with the following

A   character analysis
B   oedipal complex
C   character as an armour of the ego
D   the book 'The function of the orgasm'
E   orgone energy.

8.40   The term secondary gain as used by Sigmund Freud includes

A   receiving gifts
B   reduced conflict
C   financial compensation
D   release from responsibility
E   gaining attention.

8.41 Recognized causes of severe mental retardation include

A   toxaemia of pregnancy
B   phenylketonuria
C   Down's syndrome
D   Cri du chat syndrome
E   Turner's syndrome.

8.42 Features of anorexia nervosa include

A   amenorrhoea
B   it only occurs in females
C   it is more common in social class V
D   the TSH level is usually abnormal
E   hypotension.

8.43 Features of chronic alcoholism include

A   Marchiafava–Bignami syndrome
B   optic atrophy
C   Campbell de Morgan spots
D   episodic hypoglycaemia
E   haemochromatosis.

8.44 Class B drugs under the Misuse of Drugs Act (1971) include

A   benzphetamine
B   chlorphentermine
C   opium
D   cannabis resin
E   meprobamate.

8.45 Methadone is an analgesic which

A   is approximately as potent as morphine
B   is commonly used to replace heroin in patients dependent on heroin
C   causes suppression of coughing
D   is more sedating than morphine
E   is a Class B drug under the Misuse of Drugs Act (1971).

8.46 The following drugs are recognized causes of impaired ejaculation

A   heroin
B   methadone
C   cocaine
D   cannabis
E   alcohol.

8.47   Characteristic features of puerperal psychosis include
A   it occurs in approximately 1 in 10 000 births
B   onset is within 2 weeks of delivery
C   symptoms peak on the fourth postpartum day
D   affective symptoms
E   patients recover fully.

8.48   The stop–start procedure
A   was advanced by Semans
B   is helpful for treating erectile impotence
C   involves sensate focus exercises
D   involves manual stimulation of the penis
E   is helpful for treating premature ejaculation.

8.49   Recognized treatments for obsessive–compulsive neurosis include
A   systematic desensitization
B   flooding
C   overcorrection
D   biofeedback
E   response prevention.

8.50   According to Beck, cognitive elements that maintain depression include
A   obsessions
B   magnification
C   arbitrary inference
D   psychic fragmentation
E   selective attention.

PAPER 9: SHORT-ANSWER QUESTION PAPER

9.1   A 31-year-old nurse presents with five schneiderian first-rank symptoms. List five possible diagnoses.

9.2   List 10 treatable causes of dementia.

9.3   Discuss briefly disorders of sexual object that may be seen in male patients.

9.4   List eight possible negative side-effects of psychotherapy.

9.5   List six common causes of insomnia.

9.6   Outline factors in
a.   the previous history;
b.   the mental state
     that may be associated with dangerousness.

9.7   List five short-term side-effects of electroconvulsive therapy.

9.8   What are the characteristics of phobic disorders?
Outline the various therapeutic methods which may be used to treat a patient with a phobic disorder.

9.9   What criteria should a defendent fulfil in order to be considered fit to plead?

9.10   Name three preventable causes of mental retardation that can be diagnosed postnatally, and briefly describe details of their detection and prevention measures.

9.11   Briefly outline the factors which, following their study of depressed women in London, Brown & Harris (1978) identified as being associated with depression.

9.12   The following drugs interact with phenytoin:
   i. chlorpromazine;
   ii. carbamazepine;
   iii. lithium carbonate;
   iv. the oral contraceptive pill.
For each of the above drugs state:
  a. the mechanism of the interaction with phenytoin;
  b. a possible outcome of the interaction.

9.13   Outline the relative merits of:
  a. categories;
  b. dimensions
in psychiatric classification.

9.14   Briefly describe four sources of variation in clinical trials.

9.15   List the names given to types of waves seen in an EEG, classified by increasing frequency, starting with the lowest frequency range.
  a. Name two classes of drugs that cause fast EEG waves.
  b. Name two classes of drugs that cause slow EEG waves.

9.16   Outline the principles of the family study method for investigating genetics.
Discuss briefly two possible problems with this method and their solutions.

9.17   List
  a. two inventories;
  b. two projective tests
which can be used as psychological tests of personality.

9.18 What is meant by the term supersensitivity as used in neuropharmacology?
Outline the evidence to support the supersensitivity hypothesis for the development of tardive dyskinesia.

9.19 What is meant by the following terms:
a. incidence;
b. prevalence;
c. attributable risk?

9.20 What is the multiple correlation coefficient?
List any three assumptions that are made in its determination.

Answers

1.1 A **False** Standing with slight support usually appears at approximately 12 months
B **False** Usually appears at approximately 40 weeks
C **True** Usually appears at approximately 28 weeks
D **False** Usually appears at approximately 4 weeks and therefore has already begun
E **False** Gender identify is firmly established by about $2\frac{1}{2}$ to 3 years

Ref. Comprehensive Textbook of Psychiatry, 4th edn, pp 1599–1600

1.2 A **False** Associated with Freud
B **True** Occurs in the preoperational representation stage
C **False** Associated with Erikson
D **True** Occurs in the preoperational representation stage
E **False** Associated with Freud

Ref. Comprehensive Textbook of Psychiatry, 4th edn, pp 178–182, 360, 371

1.3 A **True**
B **True**
C **False** Associated with Piaget
D **True**
E **True**

Ref. Comprehensive Textbook of Psychiatry, 4th edn, pp 1594, 1767

1.4 A **False** This is seen in dominant parietal lobe dysfunction
B **False** This is seen in dominant temporal lobe dysfunction
C **False** This is seen in hypothalamic dysfunction
D **False** This is seen in parietal lobe dysfunction
E **False** Impaired initiative is seen

Ref. Companion to Psychiatric Studies, 4th edn, pp 257–261

1.5 A **True**
     B **False**
     C **True**   This test and the associated Role Construct Repertory Test are closely linked with the Personal Construct of Kelly

     D **False**
     E **True**

Ref. Companion to Psychiatric Studies, 4th edn, pp 236–237

1.6 A **False**   In aversion therapy an unpleasant sensation is produced in the patient
     B **False**   The treatment of choice is programmed practice
     C **True**
     D **True**
     E **False**

Ref. Companion to Psychiatric Studies, 4th edn, pp 770–771; Oxford Textbook of Psychiatry, pp 163, 604

1.7 A **False**   Neuroleptics cause slow waves
     B **False**   Tricyclic antidepressants cause slow waves
     C **True**
     D **False**
     E **True**

Ref. The Scientific Basis of Psychiatry, pp 125–126

1.8 A **False**   As they are developing they remain isolated
     B **False**   These are the responses of normally reared monkeys
     C **True**
     D **True**
     E **True**

Ref. The Scientific Basis of Psychiatry, pp 437–438

1.9 A **False**
     B **False**
     C **True**
     D **True**
     E **True**

Ref. Treatment and Management in Adult Psychiatry, pp 462–463

1.10 A **True**   Sympathetic ganglia are nicotinic
     B **False**
     C **False**
     D **False**
     E **True**

Ref. Clinical Neuroanatomy for Medical Students, 2nd edn, pp 464–466

1.11 A **False**
      B **True**
      C **False**   These will increase the actions of acetylcholine
      D **True**
      E **False**

Ref. Companion to Psychiatric Studies, 4th edn, p 122–125

1.12 A **True**
      B **False**   This is a precursor of 5-HT
      C **True**
      D **False**   Phenylalanine is a precursor
      E **True**

Ref. Companion to Psychiatric Studies, 4th edn, p 133

1.13 A **False**
      B **True**
      C **True**
      D **True**
      E **True**

Ref. Davidson's Principles and Practice of Medicine, 13th edn,
      pp 459–460

1.14 A **False**
      B **True**
      C **True**
      D **False**
      E **True**

Ref. Clinical Neuroanatomy for Medical Students, 2nd edn, pp 242–244

1.15 A **True**
      B **False**
      C **True**
      D **False**
      E **False**

Ref. Lecture Notes on Clinical Medicine, 2nd edn, p 8

1.16 A **False**   This is a metencephalic structure
      B **False**   These are telencephalic structures
      C **False**   This is a metencephalic structure
      D **True**
      E **True**

Ref. Companion to Psychiatric Studies, 4th edn, p 87

1.17 A **False**   This is a precursor of 5-HT
B **False**
C **True**
D **True**
E **True**

Ref. Companion to Psychiatric Studies, 4th edn, pp 118–121

1.18 A **False**   This is a precursor of histamine
B **False**
C **False**   Serotonin is 5-hydroxytryptamine
D **False**   This is a precursor of DOPA
E **False**   5-hydroxyindolacetic acid is formed by the
catabolism of serotonin by monoamine oxidase

Ref. Companion to Psychiatric Studies, 4th edn, p 121–122

1.19 A **True**
B **False**   Noradrenaline not dopamine
C **True**
D **False**   5-HT not adrenalin
E **False**

Ref. Companion to Psychiatric Studies, 4th edn, chapter 7

1.20 A **True**
B **False**
C **False**
D **True**
E **True**

Ref. Companion to Psychiatric Studies, 3rd edn, p 145

1.21 **All true**

Ref. The Scientific Basis of Psychiatry, chapter 13;
British National Formulary, number 15, pp 143–144

1.22 A **False**
B **True**
C **True**
D **True**
E **True**

Ref. The Scientific Basis of Psychiatry, pp 230–231

1.23 A **False**
B **False**
C **True**
D **True**
E **True**

Ref. Companion to Psychiatric Studies, 4th edn, pp 126–128

1.24 A **True**   In the case of mianserin it is recommended that a full
blood count is carried out every 4 weeks during the
first 3 months of treatment
B **False**   There are fewer and milder anticholinergic side-
effects with mianserin compared with amitriptyline
C **True**
D **False**   There are fewer and milder cardiovascular effects
with mianserin compared with amitriptyline
E **False**

Ref. British National Formulary, number 15, pp 152–153, 155

1.25 A **False**   Anorexia is a side-effect
B **False**   Amphetamines have no place in the management of
depression
C **True**
D **False**
E **True**

Ref. British National Formulary, number 15, p 159

1.26 A **False**   This is a beta-adrenoceptor blocker
B **True**
C **True**
D **True**
E **True**

Ref. British National Formulary, number 15 pp 354, 437

1.27 A **False**   The term was coined by Barton
B **False**   Inability to plan for the future
C **False**   Barton considered it to be a 'disease' which was
independent of the original illness on admission
D **True**
E **True**

Ref. Companion to Psychiatric Studies, 4th edn, p 21

1.28 A **True**
B **True**
C **False**
D **False**
E **True**

Ref. Companion to Psychiatric Studies, 4th edn, pp 20–21;
Goffman E 1968 Asylums. Penguin, London

1.29 All true

Ref. Companion to Psychiatric Studies, 4th edn, p 215

1.30 A **True**
B **False**
C **True**
D **True**
E **False**

Ref. Companion to Psychiatric Studies, 3rd edn, p 24;
Karl S B, Cobb S 1986 Health behaviour, illness behaviour and sick-role behaviour. Archives of Environmental Health 12: 246–266

1.31 A **False**   This is the simple 'legal' family, a couple with one or more children
B **True**
C **True**
D **False**   This is the same as A above
E **False**   This comprises the rules prohibiting marriage with a person who is a member of the group one belongs to

Ref. Basic Sociology, 4th ed, pp 69–70

1.32 All true

Ref. Basic Sociology, 4th edn, pp 86–93

1.33 A **True**
B **True**
C **True**
D **True**
E **False**

Ref. Companion to Psychiatric Studies, 4th edn, chapter 9;
The Scientific Basis of Psychiatry, chapter 16

1.34 A **False**
B **True**
C **False**
D **True**
E **True**

Ref. Companion to Psychiatric Studies, 4th edn, chapter 9;
Comprehensive Textbook of Psychiatry, 4th edn, p 1647;
The Scientific Basis of Psychiatry, chapter 16

1.35 A **True**
B **True**
C **False**
D **True**
E **True**

Ref. Companion to Psychiatric Studies, 4th edn, chapter 9;
The Scientific Basis of Psychiatry, chapter 16

1.36 A **True**
 B **True**
 C **True**
 D **True**
 E **False**

> **Ref.** Companion to Psychiatric Studies, 4th edn, chapter 9;
> The Scientific Basis of Psychiatry, chapter 16;
> Davidson's Principles and Practice of Medicine, 13th edn, p 16

1.37 A **False**   It only occurs in males
 B **False**
 C **True**   There is more than one X chromosome
 D **True**
 E **True**

> **Ref.** Companion to Psychiatric Studies, 4th edn, pp 161, 185, 443

1.38 All true

> **Ref.** Oxford Textbook of Psychiatry, p 68

1.39 A **True**   Lewis suggested that illness could be characterized
     by evident disturbance of part functions as well as
     general efficiency
 B **False**
 C **True**
 D **True**
 E **True**

> **Ref.** Oxford Textbook of Psychiatry, p 69

1.40 A **True**
 B **False**
 C **False**
 D **True**
 E **False**

> **Ref.** Oxford Textbook of Psychiatry, pp 73–75

1.41 A **False**
 B **True**
 C **True**
 D **True**
 E **False**   Goldberg & Huxley found that in general family
     doctors detect emotional disorders more readily
     among women, the separated, the widowed, and the
     middle-aged

> **Ref.** Oxford Textbook of Psychiatry, pp 137–138

1.42 A **False**
       B **False**
       C **False**
       D **False**
       E **True**

Ref. Oxford Textbook of Psychiatry, p 400

1.43 A **False**
       B **False**
       C **False**
       D **True**
       E **True**

Ref. Oxford Textbook of Psychiatry, p 411

1.44 A **True**
       B **False**
       C **True**
       D **True**
       E **True**

Ref. Oxford Textbook of Psychiatry, pp 442–443

1.45 A **True**
       B **True**
       C **True**
       D **False**
       E **False**

Ref. Companion to Psychiatric Studies, 2nd edn, pp 217–218

1.46 A **False**
       B **True**
       C **False**   The standard deviation is the square root of the
                   variance and therefore it follows that when the value
                   of the variance is greater than zero and less than one,
                   the standard deviation will be greater than the
                   variance
       D **True**
       E **False**   The mean will be greater than the median in such a
                   distribution

Ref. Companion to Psychiatric Studies, 2nd edn, chapter 14

1.47 A **True**
B **True**
C **False**   Let the standard error of the mean be x. Then the 95% confidence limits for the mean will given by the range [(mean) + 1.96x] to [(mean) − 1.96x]. This equals 5 − 1 (given in the question) which is 4. Hence it follows that $4x = 4$, whence $x = 1$ (approximately)
D **False**   Because 4.75 lies within the 95% confidence limits
E **False**

Ref. Companion to Psychiatric Studies, 2nd edn, chapter 14; Statistics at Square One, chapter 4

1.48 All false

Ref. Companion to Psychiatric Studies, 2nd edn, chapter 14

1.49 A **False**
B **False**
C **False**
D **False**
E **True**

Ref. Companion to Psychiatric Studies, 2nd edn, chapter 14

1.50 All true

Ref. Statistics at Square One, chapter 9

PAPER 2: MULTIPLE CHOICE QUESTIONS ON CLINICAL TOPICS

2.1 All true

Ref. Oxford Textbook of Psychiatry, pp 295–296

2.2 A **False**   It is transmitted by an infective agent, often referred to as a 'slow virus'.
B **True**
C **False**   Kuru is pathologically similar
D **True**
E **True**

Ref. Oxford Textbook of Psychiatry, p 314

2.3 A **True**
B **False**   Neurotic symptoms were found by Lishman not to be related to the amount of damage
C **True**
D **True**
E **True**

Ref. Oxford Textbook of Psychiatry, p 316

2.4 All true

Ref. Brain's Diseases of the Nervous System, 8th edn, p 854;
Oxford Textbook of Psychiatry, p 332

2.5 A **True**   Naloxone acts as an antidote to the
dextropropoxyphene in co-proxamol
B **True**
C **True**
D **False**   The initial features are those of acute opioid
overdosage, including pinpoint pupils
E **True**

Ref. British National Formulary, number 15, p 38

2.6 A **False**
B **True**
C **False**
D **True**
E **False**

Ref. Oxford Textbook of Psychiatry, pp 335–336

2.7 A **True**
B **False**   The obstruction is in the subarachnoid space
C **True**
D **True**
E **False**

Ref. Companion to Psychiatric Studies, 4th edn, pp 292–293
Companion to Psychiatric Studies, 3rd edn, p 272;
Oxford Textbook of Psychiatry, pp 314–315

2.8 A **True**
B **True**
C **True**
D **False**   The parents characteristically persist in maintaining
that the injuries are accidental
E **False**   An alert but inhibited appearance may be exhibited,
known as 'frozen watchfulness'

Ref. Oxford Textbook of Psychiatry, pp 672–673

2.9 A **False**   Conduct disorders are the most frequent psychiatric
disorders of childhood
B **False**   Rutter et al (1970) found a prevalence of 2.5% in both
boys and girls aged 10 and 11
C **False**
D **False**
E **True**

Ref. Oxford Textbook of Psychiatry, p 646

2.10 All true

Ref. Oxford Textbook of Psychiatry, p 649

2.11 A **True**
B **True**
C **False**   Prolonged motor overactivity occurs
D **True**
E **True**

Ref. Oxford Textbook of Psychiatry, pp 657–658

2.12 A **False**   This is a DSM-III R category — 301.60
B **False**   This is a DSM-III R category — 301.22
C **False**   This is a DSM-III R category — 301.50
D **False**   This is a DSM-III R category — 301.40
E **True**   301.2

Ref. Mental Disorders: Glossary and Guide to their Classification in Accordance with the Ninth Revision of the International Classification of Diseases;
Diagnostic and Statistical Manual of Mental Disorders, 3rd Edn — revised;
Oxford Textbook of Psychiatry p 110

2.13 A **False**   Described by Sheldon et al (1940, 1942)
B **False**   Described by Sheldon et al (1940, 1942)
C **False**   Described by Sheldon et al (1940, 1942)
D **False**   Described by Sheldon et al (1940, 1942)
E **False**

Ref. Oxford Textbook of Psychiatry, p 119

2.14 A **True**
B **False**   There is a moderate genetic influence
C **True**
D **True**
E **False**

Ref. Oxford Textbook of Psychiatry, pp 140–148

2.15 A **True**
B **True**
C **False**
D **True**
E **True**

Ref. Oxford Textbook of Psychiatry, pp 157–159

2.16 All true

Ref. Oxford Textbook of Psychiatry, pp 110–111

2.17 A **True**   This is an early reaction to bereavement
    B **False**
    C **False**
    D **False**
    E **True**

Ref. Handbook of Affective Disorders, pp 403, 405;
    Oxford Textbook of Psychiatry, p 194

2.18 A **False**   It was propounded by Seligman
    B **True**
    C **True**
    D **False**   Decreased voluntary activity is a characteristic
        feature
    E **True**

Ref. Handbook of Affective Disorders, pp 203–204;
    Oxford Textbook of Psychiatry, pp 208–209;
    Companion to Psychiatric Studies, 4th edn, pp 130, 409

2.19 A **True**
    B **False**   The only treatment is tooth-protectors
    C **True**
    D **True**
    E **True**   It may lead to damage to the teeth

Ref. Treatment and Management in Adult Psychiatry, pp 472–473

2.20 A **False**
    B **True**
    C **False**
    D **False**
    E **False**

Ref. Oxford Textbook of Psychiatry, p 237;
    Companion to Psychiatric Studies, 4th edn, p 312

2.21 A **False**
    B **True**
    C **True**
    D **False**   The category of younger depressive with personality
        disorder was described by Paykel
    E **True**

Ref. Paykel ES 1971 Classification of depressed patients: a cluster
    analysis derived grouping. British Journal of Psychiatry 118;
    275–288;
    Handbook of Affective Disorders, pp 38–40, 86

2.22 A **True**
B **False**
C **False**   It was described by Kral (1962)
D **False**   Patients are said to have difficulty in remembering; this is not progressive
E **False**   Life expectancy is unchanged

Ref. Comprehensive Textbook of Psychiatry, 4th edn, p 853;
Oxford Textbook of Psychiatry, p 507

2.23 A **False**   Its onset is usually rapid
B **False**   It is more common in males
C **True**   Fits are common
D **True**   Depressive symptoms are common
E **True**

Ref. Oxford Textbook of Psychiatry, pp 508–509;
Companion to Psychiatric Studies, 4th edn, pp 283–284, 576

2.24 A **True**
B **False**   The figure is approximately 15%
C **False**
D **False**
E **False**

Ref. Companion to Psychiatric Studies, 4th edn, pp 464–465

2.25 A **True**
B **True**
C **False**
D **True**
E **True**

Ref. Oxford Textbook of Psychiatry, pp 347–348

2.26 A **False**   M : F equals approximately 2 : 1
B **False**   The rates of all types of psychiatric disorder in the inner London borough were approximately twice those in the Isle of Wight
C **False**   8%: this figure increased to 20% if children who expressed less severe anxiety and depression were included
D **True**
E **False**   Depressive disorders of the adult type seldom occur before puberty

Ref. Oxford Textbook of Psychiatry, pp 631–632, 648–649

2.27 A **False**   This is present in the milk in amounts too small to be harmful
B **False**   This is present in the milk in amounts too small to be harmful
C **True**   It may cause withdrawal symptoms in the infant; breast feeding is permissible during maintenance dosage
D **True**   It is important to monitor the infant for possible intoxication; good control of maternal plasma lithium levels minimizes the risk to the infant
E **True**   Significant amounts are excreted into the milk and this drug is therefore best avoided in breastfeeding mothers

Ref. British National Formulary, number 15, pp 31–33

2.28 A **False**   It is a piperazine compound
B **True**
C **False**   They are generally more sedating than piperazine compounds
D **False**   Haloperidol is a butyrophenone, not a phenothiazine
E **True**   Cf. trifluoperazine vs. thioridazine. Piperidine compounds generally have marked anticholinergic effects

Ref. Oxford Textbook of Psychiatry, pp 533–535;
British National Formulary, number 15, pp 143–144

2.29 A **False**   It is now generally agreed that there are no indications for this operation (as described by Freeman & Watts 1942). During the 3 years from 1974 to 1976, no neurosurgical operations were performed for sexual psychopathology in the British Isles (Barraclough & Mitchell-Heggs 1978)
B **True**   This is in order to minimize the risk of damaging the motor system
C **False**   This operation may be effective in treating pain caused by breast or prostatic carcinoma, but it is inappropriate for treating psychogenic pain
D **True**
E **True**   This procedure was developed at St George's Hospital, London. The operation aims to interrupt two frontolimbic pathways

Ref. Treatment and Management in Adult Psychiatry, pp 150–161;
Companion to Psychiatric Studies, 4th edn, p 722;
Oxford Textbook of Psychiatry, pp 572–573

2.30 **All true**   These are all short-term side effects of ECT

Ref. Treatment and Management in Adult Psychiatry, p 139

2.31 A **True**   He described this condition (Kanner 1943)
      B **True**
      C **False**   In 1856 Connolly published 'The treatment of the
              insane without medical restraints'
      D **True**
      E **True**

Ref. Oxford Textbook of Psychiatry, pp 659–661

2.32 A **False**   Associated with lithium therapy
      B **True**   Meduna produced fits using intramuscular camphor
              in 1934
      C **False**   Associated with work on personality
      D **True**   Produced fits by passing an electric current through
              the brain (Cerletti & Bini 1938)
      E **True**   Produced fits by passing an electric current through
              the brain (Cerletti & Bini 1938)

Ref. Oxford Textbook of Psychiatry, p 563;
      Comprehensive Textbook of Psychiatry, 4th edn, p 1558

2.33 A **False**
      B **True**   Their deaths usually result from 'abnormal' homicide
              or repeated child abuse
      C **True**
      D **True**   A large proportion of murderers are under the
              influence of alcohol at the time of the crime
      E **True**

Ref. Oxford Textbook of Psychiatry, pp 723, 731–732

2.34 A **True**
      B **True**
      C **False**   It is criminal law and not civil law which is concerned
              with offences against the state
      D **True**
      E **True**

Ref. Oxford Textbook of Psychiatry, pp 717–719

2.35 A **True**
      B **False**   The victims are known to the offender in four-fifths of
              cases, and belong to the offender's family in one-
              third of cases
      C **False**   Female : male is approximately 2 : 1
      D **False**   It is low
      E **True**

Ref. Oxford Textbook of Psychiatry, pp 734–735

2.36 A **True**
    B **False**   Associated with Carl G. Jung
    C **False**   Associated with Alfred Adler
    D **True**
    E **False**   Associated with Carl G. Jung

    Ref. Comprehensive Textbook of Psychiatry, 4th edn, pp 345–346, 348, 436, 453

2.37 A **True**
    B **False**   This is a major approach to inner harmony
    C **False**   This is a major approach to inner harmony
    D **True**
    E **True**   Also known as compartmentalization

    Ref. Comprehensive Textbook of Psychiatry, 4th edn, pp 420–424

2.38 A **False**   Associated with C. G. Jung
    B **False**   Associated with H. S. Sullivan
    C **True**
    D **False**   Associated with E. Erikson
    E **True**

    Ref. Comprehensive Textbook of Psychiatry, 4th edn, pp 429, 435, 453–454

2.39 A **False**   Client-centred psychotherapy is associated with Rogers
    B **True**
    C **True**
    D **False**   Bioenergetics is associated with Reich
    E **True**

    Ref. Comprehensive Textbook of Psychiatry, 4th edn, pp 446, 455–456, 1374, 1457

2.40 A **False**   This has not been reported in homocystinuria (although it is a recognized feature of Marfan's syndrome)
    B **True**
    C **True**
    D **False**   This is reduced
    E **True**

    Ref. Metabolic Control and Disease, 8th edn, p 667

2.41 A **False**   It is more common in males
    B **True**
    C **False**   It is usually mild or moderate
    D **True**
    E **True**   These may be seen on the iris

    Ref. Oxford Textbook of Psychiatry, pp 700–701;
    Companion to Psychiatric Studies, 4th edn, pp 441–442

2.42 A **True**
B **True**
C **False** Not caused by a virus
D **False** Not caused by a virus
E **False** This is neither a recognized cause of mental retardation nor is this disease caused by a virus

Ref. Oxford Textbook of Psychiatry, p 695

2.43 A **True** 10–20% admit to stealing food, including by shoplifting
B **True**
C **False** The peak onset is at approximately age 12 in males
D **False**
E **True**

Ref. Oxford Textbook of Psychiatry, pp 365–368

2.44 A **True**
B **True**
C **False** Hypokalaemia is common
D **False** Dilatation of the pupils usually occurs
E **True**

Ref. Oxford Textbook of Psychiatry, p 427;
Companion to Psychiatric Studies, 4th edn, pp 262–263

2.45 A **True**
B **True**
C **True**
D **True**
E **False** Oral amphetamines are included under class B.

Ref. British National Formulary, number 15, p 8

2.46 A **True**
B **False** Only approximately 5% are solitary abusers
C **True**
D **False** There is no specific treatment for solvent abuse
E **False** Hallucinations are mainly visual

Ref. Oxford Textbook of Psychiatry, pp 454–455

2.47 A **False** More common in males
B **True**
C **True**
D **True**
E **True**

Ref. Comprehensive Textbook of Psychiatry, 4th edn, p 1086

2.48 **All true**

Ref. Comprehensive Textbook of Psychiatry, 4th edn, p 1174

2.49 A **False**   This occurs in aversion therapy
     B **True**
     C **False**
     D **False**   This involves exposure to the stimulus in a non-graded manner with no attempt to reduce anxiety
     E **True**   The method most often used is that developed by Jacobson

Ref. Companion to Psychiatric Studies, 4th edn, pp 769–770

2.50 A **False**
     B **True**   It is usually used in conjunction with other techniques such as flooding
     C **True**   It is usually used in conjunction with other techniques such as flooding
     D **True**
     E **True**

Ref. Companion to Psychiatric Studies, 4th edn, p 772

PAPER 3 SHORT-ANSWER QUESTION PAPER

3.1   a. Carcinoma; infections; side-effects of drugs; diabetes; hypothyroidism; hyperparathyroidism, systemic lupus erythematosus; Addison's disease/hypoadrenalism; dementias; etc. (give any five)
     b. Epilepsy; hypoglycaemia; phaeochromocytoma; metabolic disorders e.g. uraemia, acute intermittent porphyria; transient global amnesia; early dementia; etc. (give any five)

Ref. Oxford Textbook of Psychiatry, pp 200–201, 326–327, 330, 337, 352

3.2   a. G. F. M. Russell (1979).
     b. An intractable urge to overeat; self-induced vomiting and/or abuse of laxatives; a morbid fear of becoming fat; (give any two)
     c. Hypothalamic tumours;
       Klein–Levin syndrome

Ref. Oxford Textbook of Psychiatry, pp 370–371;
      Russell G 1979 Psychological Medicine 9: 429–448

3.3   Repeated involuntary voiding of urine during sleep, after an age
at which continence is expected. Not caused by a physical
disorder.
Measures:
- First step is to exclude a physical disorder (the question does
  not state it is a case of functional nocturnal enuresis), e.g. a
  urinary tract infection, diabetes, or a neurological disorder
  such as epilepsy
- Look for and treat any psychiatric disorder present
- Family assessment and family therapy where appropriate
- Enuresis alarm method (bell and pad): one-third relapse
- Star chart
- Tricyclic antidepressant medication (but high relapse rate
  when stopped, side-effects, and danger of overdose)

Ref. Oxford Textbook of Psychiatry, pp 668–670

3.4   Autosomal recessive inborn error of metabolism
Deficiency of cystathionine synthetase leads to increased
homocystine and increased methionine
Clinical features include: fine and fair hair, ectopia lentis,
skeletal abnormalities, epilepsy, mental retardation,
thromboembolic episodes, etc.
Heterozygotes may be detected by methionine loading
Sometimes can be treated with methionine-free diet

Ref. Oxford Textbook of Psychiatry, p 696;
Companion to Psychiatric Studies, 4th edn, p 149

3.5   Altruism
Catharsis
Corrective recapitulation of primary family group
Development of socializing techniques
Existential awareness
Group cohesiveness
Guidance
Imitative behaviour
Insight
Instillation of hope
Interpersonal learning
Universality

Ref. Yalom I D 1975 The theory and practice of group psychotherapy,
2nd edn. New York, Basic Books

3.6   **Amok** — SE Asia — Outburst of aggressive behaviour following an episode of depression. May end with the person killing himself or being killed, often after killing others himself
Koro — SE Asia, China — Occurs in men. Fear of penis retracting into abdomen and of imminent death subsequent to this
Latah — Far East — Hysterical state with echolalia, echopraxia, and automatic obedience
Piblokto — Eskimo women — Dissociative state. May lead to murder or suicide
Susto/Espanto — High Andes — Prolonged depressive state believed by sufferers to be caused by supernatural agencies
Windigo — N. American Indian tribes — Sufferers believe they have mutated into cannabalistic monsters
(Give any five)

Ref.   Comprehensive Textbook of Psychiatry 4th edn, pp 256–258;
       Companion to Psychiatric Studies, 2nd edn, p 26;
       Oxford Textbook of Psychiatry, p 175

3.7   **Causes**
Thiamine deficiency (caused by e.g. chronic alcohol abuse, nutritional insufficiency, malabsorption, intractable vomiting)
Carbon monoxide poisoning
Head injury
Heavy metal poisoning
Third ventricle tumours
Bilateral hippocampal damage e.g. surgical
Anaesthetic accidents
(Give any five)
Clinical features
Disorientation
Impaired recent memory
Confabulation
Apathy and diminished drive
(Give any three)

Ref.   Oxford Textbook of Psychiatry, pp 299–301;
       Mental Disorders Glossary and Guide to their classification in
       Accordance with the Ninth Revision of the International
       Classification of Diseases;
       Companion to Psychiatric Studies, 4th edn, p 248

3.8 Dementia is a generalized impairment of intellect, memory and personality in clear consciousness. Most cases of dementia are irreversible, although a small group are remediable.
Clinical features — Usually insidious onset, but may come to notice following an illness or change in social circumstances. Impaired recent memory. Frontal, temporal and parietal lobe dysfunction. Speech disorders, e.g. nominal dysphasias and sometimes eventually muteness or meaningless noises. Disinhibition. Apathy. Agitation. Mood changes. Incontinence. Epilepsy

Ref. Oxford Textbook of Psychiatry, pp 297–299

3.9 **Factors** — The nature of the illness and its significance to the patient. The effect of the illness on social and occupational functioning. Advantages of the sick role. Patient traits
Patterns of response
Denial — can be a useful defence mechanism against overwhelming anxiety, but may cause a delay in seeking treatment
Coping — coping strategies include seeking information and social withdrawal
Social adjustment
Prolongation of the sick role — for secondary gain
Paranoid reaction — may blame doctor
Depression
Preoccupation with illness

Ref. Oxford Textbook of Psychiatry, pp 353–354
Lloyd CG 1977 Psychological reactions to physical illness. British Journal of Hospital Medicine 18: 352–358

3.10 Previous deliberate self-harm
Previous psychiatric treatment (both inpatient and outpatient)
Personality disorder
Alcohol abuse
Drug abuse
Criminal record
Low social class
Unemployment

Ref. Kreitman N et al. 1980 Suicide in relation to parasuicide. Medicine (3rd series) 36: 1830;
Oxford Textbook of Psychiatry, pp 416–417

3.11 The validity of a test is the degree to which a test measures what it is meant to measure, whereas the reliability of a test is the consistency with which the test obtains the results
Types of validity
Content/sampling validity
Predictive validity
Construct validity
Criterion validity
Face validity
Procedural validity
(Give any three)
Types of reliability
Inter-rater reliability
Test–retest reliability
Alternate-form reliability
Split-half reliability
(Give any three)

Ref. Comprehensive Textbook of Psychiatry, 4th edn, pp 299–300;
    Companion to Psychiatric Studies, 4th edn, pp 219–221, 224–226

3.12 Diagnoses in psychiatry often convey little or no information about aetiology, symptomatology, treatment or prognosis
Most patients do not fit neatly into textbook categories
Psychiatric diagnoses may have pejorative connotations
They give the false impression of a greater understanding of a disease than may exist
The reliability and validity levels of psychiatric diagnoses are low
Applying psychiatric diagnostic labels may lead to the clinician no longer viewing patients as unique individuals

Ref. Companion to Psychiatric Studies, 4th edn, p 208

3.13   In an autosomal dominant condition the effect of the autosomal dominant gene is seen in a subject carrying the gene in a single or double dose, i.e. in the heterozygous or homozygous form, whereas in an autosomal recessive condition the effect of the autosomal recessive gene is seen only when the gene is present in the double dose of the homozygous form. Sex-linked inheritance is present when the gene coding for the disorder or trait is carried on the X chromosome. (It may be helpful to add clear, well drawn diagrams.)

Autosomal dominant — tuberous sclerosis; von Recklinghausen's disease (neurofibromatosis); Sturge–Weber syndrome; etc. (give any two)

Autosomal recessive — phenylketonuria; homocystinuria; maple syrup disease; etc. (give any two)

Sex-linked — Hunter's syndrome; Lesch–Nyhan syndrome (hyperuricaemia); oculocerebrorenal syndrome of Lowe; etc. (give any two)

Ref.   Companion to Psychiatric Studies, 4th edn. pp 163, 183–187
Comprehensive Textbook of Psychiatry, 4th edn, pp 26–28, 1647

3.14   L-tyrosine: hydroxylated by tyrosine hydroxylase to L-dopa
L-dopa: decarboxylated by L-dopa decarboxylase (= L-aromatic amino acid decarboxylase) to dopamine
Dopamine: hydoxylated by dopamine β-hydroxylase to noradrenaline
Inhibitors
Tyrosine hydroxylase: α-methyl-p-tyrosine
Dopa decarboxylase: carbidopa
Dopamine β-hydroxylase: disulfiram

Ref.   Companion to Psychiatric Studies, 4th edn, p 133

3.15   **Anterior lobe**
Adrenocorticotrophic hormone/corticotrophin
Melanocyte-stimulating hormone
Luteinizing hormone
Follicle-stimulating hormone
Growth hormone/somatotrophin
Thyroid-stimulating hormone/thyrotrophin
Prolactin
Posterior lobe
Oxytocin — paraventricular nuclei
Vasopressin/antidiuretic hormone — supraoptic nuclei

Ref.   Davidson's Principles and Practice of Medicine, 13th edn, pp 459–460

SWANSEA PSYCHIATRIC EDUCATION LIBRARY

3.16   The trochlear nerve (cranial nerve IV) innervates the superior oblique muscle. The abducent nerve (cranial nerve VI) innervates the lateral rectus muscle. The oculomotor nerve (cranial nerve III) innervates all the remaining extrinsic muscles of the eye, i.e. the superior rectus muscle, the inferior rectus muscle, the medial rectus muscle and the inferior oblique muscle.
VI nerve palsy — leads to failure of lateral movement with convergent strabismus. Diplopia maximal when looking to the affected side, leading to parallel and horizontally separated images.
IV nerve palsy — leads to diplopia maximal when looking downwards.
III nerve palsy — leads to ptosis; eye is 'down and out' (divergent strabismus); severe diplopia; pupil dilated (because of interference with the parasympathetic supply).

Ref. Lecture Notes on Clinical Medicine, 2nd edn, pp 7–8;
    Clinical Neuroanatomy for Medical Students, 2nd edn, p 427

3.17   **1.** Benzodiazepines are much safer than barbiturates in overdose
2. Whilst benzodiazepines may cause physical dependence with chronic use, barbiturates have a much higher tendency to cause the development of both psychological and physical dependence
3. Benzodiazepines generally tend not to cause the induction of hepatic microsomal enzymes, whilst the opposite is true of barbiturates. This causes the latter to alter the metabolism of other drugs such as steroids and anticoagulant medication
Side-effects
Drowsiness
Confusion
Ataxia
Dizziness
Release of aggression
Dry mouth
Headaches
Hypersensitivity reactions
Respiratory depression
(give any seven)

Ref. Treatment and Management in Adult Psychiatry, pp 3–11;
    British National Formulary, number 15, pp 135–142

3.18   **Aged 0–2 years:** Sensorimotor stage
- distinguishes himself/herself from the environment
- object constancy and object permanence

Aged 2–7 years: Preoperational representation stage
- egocentrism
- animism
- precausal reasoning
- authoritarian morality

Aged 7–12 years: Concrete operational stage
- laws of conservation (e.g. of volume)

Aged over 12 years: Formal operational stage
- abstract thought

Ref. Comprehensive Textbook of Psychiatry, 4th edn, pp 179–183

3.19   **Features**
Diffuse rigidity of the muscles ± extrapyramidal signs
Change in consciousness — either stupor or coma
Sudden pyrexia
Sweating
Tachycardia
Sudden falls in blood pressure
Occasionally dyspnoea
Enzyme change
Serum creatinine phosphokinase is elevated

Ref. Kellam AMP 1987 British Journal of Psychiatry 150: 752–759

3.20   The intelligence quotient gives an index of intelligence, as the ratio of the mental age obtained on testing to the chronological age, expressed as a percentage.

Stanford–Binet Scale
Wechsler Adult Intelligence Scale
Wechsler Intelligence Scale for Children
(give any two)

Wechsler Adult Intelligence Scale
    Verbal scale:
        Information
        Comprehension
        Digit span
        Arithmetic
        Similarities
        Vocabulary
    Performance scale:
        Digit symbol
        Picture completion
        Block design
        Picture arrangement
        Object assembly
        (give any five)

Ref. Introduction to Psychology, 8th edn, pp 355–360

PAPER 4: MULTIPLE CHOICE QUESTIONS ON BASIC SCIENCES

4.1 A **False**   Described by Freud
    B **True**
    C **False**   Described by Freud
    D **False**   Freud described the Electra complex
    E **True**

Ref. Comprehensive Textbook of Psychiatry, 4th edn, pp 179–183

4.2 A **False**
    B **False**
    C **True**
    D **True**
    E **True**

Ref. Comprehensive Textbook of Psychiatry, 4th edn, pp 1034–1035

4.3 A **True**   Freud initially gave this as the female equivalent of
                the Oedipus complex, but later the latter term came
                to be used for this stage of psychosexual
                development in both sexes
    B **False**   Described by Piaget
    C **True**
    D **False**
    E **False**   Jung described the process of individuation as the
                growth of personality that occurs by becoming what
                one is intrinsically

Ref. Comprehensive Textbook of Psychiatry, 4th edn, pp 359–362

4.4 A **True**
    B **True**
    C **False**
    D **True**
    E **True**

Ref. The Scientific Basis of Psychiatry, p 440

4.5 A **False**   A strict hierarchical presentation of phobic items is
                not necessary
    B **True**
    C **True**
    D **True**
    E **False**

Ref. Companion to Psychiatric Studies, 4th edn, pp 769–770

4.6 A **True**
      B **True**
      C **True**
      D **True**
      E **False**   Bowlby did some important work on maternal deprivation in humans

Ref. The Scientific Basis of Psychiatry, pp 436–437

4.7 A **False**   Seen in temporal lobe dysfunction
      B **True**
      C **True**
      D **False**   Seen in dominant temporal lobe dysfunction
      E **False**

Ref. Companion to Psychiatric Studies, 4th edn, p 259–261

4.8 All false

Ref. Treatment and Management in Adult Psychiatry, pp 462–464

4.9 A **False**   Dilatation of the pupil is an α effect
      B **False**   Dilatation of the pupil is an α effect
      C **False**   Diamorphine causes pupil constriction
      D **True**
      E **True**   Adrenaline acts on both α and β receptors

4.10 A **True**
       B **True**
       C **False**   Noradrenaline is an intermediate in the biosynthesis of adrenaline.
       D **False**
       E **False**

Ref. Companion to Psychiatric Studies, 4th edn, p 115

4.11 A **True**
       B **True**
       C **False**   Benzodiazepines cause fast activity
       D **True**
       E **False**

Ref. The Scientific Basis of Psychiatry, pp 125–126

4.12 A **False**   This is an anterior pituitary hormone
       B **True**   This is vasopressin
       C **False**   This is growth hormone, which is an anterior pituitary hormone
       D **True**   This is another name for the antidiuretic hormone, as in part B above
       E **True**

Ref. Davidson's Principles and Practice of Medicine, 13th edn, pp 459–460

4.13 A **True**
    B **True**
    C **False**
    D **True**
    E **True**

    Ref. Companion to Psychiatric Studies, 4th edn, chapter 6 and 7

4.14 A **False**
    B **False**
    C **True**
    D **True**
    E **True**

    Ref. Companion to Psychiatric Studies, 3rd edn, p 179

4.15 A **True**
    B **True**
    C **False**   Less than 2% of the total body 5-HT is in the central nervous system
    D **True**
    E **True**

    Ref. Companion to Psychiatric Studies, 4th edn, pp 121–122

4.16 A **False**   This is a precursor of the neurotransmitter 5-HT
    B **True**   The locus coeruleus is in the pons
    C **False**   Homovanillic acid is a breakdown product of dopamine
    D **True**
    E **True**

    Ref. Companion to Psychiatric Studies, 4th edn, pp 115–117

4.17 A **True**
    B **True**
    C **True**
    D **False**
    E **False**

    Ref. Companion to Psychiatric Studies, 4th edn, p 96

4.18 A **False**
    B **False**
    C **False**
    D **True**
    E **False**

    Ref. Companion to Psychiatric Studies, 4th edn, p 125

4.19 A **False**
     B **True**
     C **True**
     D **False**
     E **False**   Lithium is an element (present in the form of positively charged cations in the plasma) and is not metabolized

Ref. Companion to Psychiatric Studies, 4th edn, chapter 7

4.20 A **False**
     B **False**
     C **False**   They are probably involved in respiratory stimulation not depression

     D **True**
     E **True**

Ref. Companion to Psychiatric Studies, 3rd edn, p 145

4.21 A **True**
     B **True**
     C **False**   Prolonged ventricular repolarization is a recognized neuroleptic side-effect

     D **True**
     E **False**   Constipation may occur, as an anticholinergic side-effect

Ref. The Scientific Basis of Psychiatry, chapter 13;
     British National Formulary, number 15, pp 143–145

4.22 A **False**
     B **False**   It has fewer anticholinergic effects
     C **False**
     D **True**
     E **False**   Extrapyramidal symptoms, particularly dystonic reactions and akathisia are more frequent, especially in hyperthyroidism

Ref. The Scientific Basis of Psychiatry, chapter 13;
     British National Formulary, number 15, p 146

4.23 A **True**
     B **True**
     C **False**   Respiratory depression
     D **True**
     E **False**   Diazepam, like certain other benzodiazepines (for example, temazepam) is sometimes prescribed for insomnia, although in general this is not a practice to be encouraged

Ref. British National Formulary, number 15, p 139

4.24 A **True**
B **False**
C **True**
D **True**
E **True**

Ref. The Scientific Basis of Psychiatry, p 194;
British National Formulary, number 15, pp 158–159

4.25 A **True**
B **False**   In general, cheese contains a significant amount of amines (especially tyramine) per unit weight so it should be avoided by patients taking monoamine oxidase inhibitors; this does not apply, however, to cottage cheese or cream cheese
C **True**
D **True**
E **True**

Ref. British National Formulary, number 15, p 157;
Treatment and Management in Adult Psychiatry, p 76

4.26 A **False**   Highest in social classes I and II
B **True**
C **True**
D **True**
E **False**

Ref. Companion to Psychiatric Studies, 4th edn, pp 461, 468, 589

4.27 A **True**
B **False**
C **True**
D **True**
E **False**

Ref. Companion to Psychiatric Studies, 3rd edn, p 17

4.28 A **True**   Erving Goffman, a sociologist, conducted a study at this hospital
B **True**   See the answer to part A above
C **True**
D **False**   These are not institutions that encompass most of the daily experience of pupils, unlike boarding schools
E **True**

Ref. Companion to Psychiatric Studies, 4th edn, p 20

4.29 A **True**
　　B **False**
　　C **True**
　　D **True**
　　E **True**

Ref. Companion to Psychiatric Studies, 4th edn, pp 215–216, 319

4.30 A **False**
　　B **False**
　　C **False**
　　D **False**
　　E **True**

Ref. Companion to Psychiatric Studies, 3rd edn, p 24

4.31 A **False**
　　B **True**
　　C **False**
　　D **True**
　　E **True**

Ref. Companion to Psychiatric Studies, 3rd edn, p 21

4.32 A **False** The number of Barr bodies is equal to one less than the number of X chromosomes in a nucleus. Thus in a normal male, with one X chromosome per non-gamete nucleus, a Barr body will not be seen
　　B **True** There are two X chromosomes per non-gamete nucleus
　　C **False** There is one X chromosome per non-gamete nucleus
　　D **True** There is more than one X chromosome per non-gamete nucleus
　　E **False**

Ref. Companion to Psychiatric Studies, 4th edn, pp 161–162

4.33 A **True**
　　B **True** This is Tay–Sachs disease
　　C **False**
　　D **True**
　　E **True**

Ref. Companion to Psychiatric Studies, 4th edn, chapter 9; The Scientific Basis of Psychiatry, chapter 16.

4.34 A **True**
　　B **False** Diploid
　　C **False** It is called meiosis
　　D **False** Haploid
　　E **False** The karyotype is 46XX

Ref. Companion to Psychiatric Studies, 4th edn, pp 161–162

4.35 A **True** There is more than one X chromosome per non-gamete nucleus in phenotypic males with Klinefelter's syndrome

  B **True** There is only one X chromosome per non-gamete nucleus in phenotypic females with Turner's syndrome

  C **False** This is caused by trisomy 13

  D **False** An autosomal recessive disorder caused by a deficiency of sphingomyelinase

  E **False** An X-linked disorder caused by a deficiency of hypoxanthine guanine phosphoribosyl transferase

 Ref. Companion to Psychiatric Studies, 4th edn, chapter 9

4.36 A **False**

  B **True**

  C **False** The concordance rate for this will be approximately 100% in both monozygotic and dizygotic twins

  D **False**

  E **False** Higher concordance rates have been found in monozygotic twins than in dizygotic twins

 Ref. Companion to Psychiatric Studies, 4th edn, chapter 9;
   The Scientific Basis of Psychiatry, chapter 14

4.37 A **True**

  B **False** It is associated with above average height

  C **True**

  D **True**

  E **False** 1 in 700 male births, not 1 in 700 total births

 Ref. Companion to Psychiatric Studies, 4th edn, pp 143–144, 147,
   150–151, 444;
   The Scientific Basis of Psychiatry, pp 257–259

4.38 All true

 Ref. Companion to Psychiatric Studies, 4th edn, pp 145–146

4.39 A **False** Szasz takes the view that illness can only be defined in terms of physical pathology

  B **False** Since most do not have demonstrable physical pathology, they are not counted as being diseases by Szasz

  C **False**

  D **True**

  E **True**

 Ref. Contemporary Issues in Schizophrenia, pp 91–101;
   Companion to Psychiatric Studies, 4th edn, pp 21–22;
   Oxford Textbook of Psychiatry, pp 68–69

4.40 A **True**   An organic psychosis
     B **True**   An organic psychosis
     C **False**   A neurosis
     D **True**
     E **True**

Ref. Oxford Textbook of Psychiatry, p 70

4.41 A **True**
     B **False**
     C **True**
     D **True**
     E **True**

Ref. Companion to Psychiatric Studies, 4th edn, pp 217–218

4.42 A **True**
     B **False**
     C **True**
     D **True**
     E **True**

Ref. Oxford Textbook of Psychiatry, p 400

4.43 All true

Ref. Oxford Textbook of Psychiatry, p 433

4.44 All false   These are found in DSM-III but not in ICD 9

Ref. Oxford Textbook of Psychiatry, p 134

4.45 A **False**   It is the area under the curve that represents
              frequency, since the latter must correspond to a class
              interval width
     B **False**
     C **False**   In a histogram frequencies are represented by
              rectangles
     D **True**
     E **False**   The total frequency is equal to the total area under
              the curve

Ref. Companion to Psychiatric Studies, 2nd edn, p 216

4.46 A **True**   In a normal distribution, the median is equal to the mean

    B **True**   Approximately 95% of scores are in the range [(mean − 2σ) to (mean + 2σ)], where σ = standard deviation. Thus the range is [(100 − 40) to (100 + 40)], which is [60 to 140].

    C **False**   This is a symmetrical distribution with 100 as the mean. Therefore the required probability is 0.5

    D **False**   Approximately 50% of scores are in the range [(mean − 2σ/3) to (mean + 2σ/3)], where σ = standard deviation

    E **False**   In a normal distribution, the mode is equal to the mean; thus in this case the mode is 100

Ref. Companion to Psychiatric Studies, 2nd edn, chapter 14

4.47 A **True**
    B **False**
    C **False**   This is a measure of central tendency
    D **True**
    E **True**

Ref. Companion to Psychiatric Studies, 2nd edn, chapter 14

4.48 A **True**
    B **True**   If randomly allocated
    C **False**
    D **True**
    E **True**

Ref. Companion to Psychiatric Studies, 2nd edn, chapter 14

4.49 A **False**
    B **True**
    C **True**
    D **False**
    E **False**

Ref. Companion to Psychiatric Studies, 2nd edn, chapter 14

4.50 A **False**   This is the range
    B **True**   The Gaussian distribution is another common name for the normal distribution
    C **False**
    D **True**
    E **False**   The standard deviation is the square root of the variance

PAPER 5: MULTIPLE CHOICE QUESTIONS ON CLINICAL TOPICS

5.1 A **False** Disorientation in time and place is an invariable and important feature
    B **True**
    C **False** It is desirable to avoid the high levels of illumination found in some intensive care units
    D **True**
    E **False**

Ref. Oxford Textbook of Psychiatry, pp 295–296, 309

5.2 A **False** Men and women are affected equally
    B **True**
    C **False** Epilepsy occurs especially in younger patients
    D **False** Insight is often retained until a late stage
    E **True**

Ref. Oxford Textbook of Psychiatry, pp 312–313;
     Companion to Psychiatric Studies, 4th edn, pp 287–290

5.3 A **False**
    B **True**
    C **False** The risk of suicide is substantially increased
    D **True** This is particularly likely after frontal lobe damage
    E **True**

Ref. Oxford Textbook of Psychiatry, p 315–317

5.4 A **True**
    B **False** Barbiturates may precipitate acute porphyria attacks
    C **True**
    D **True**
    E **False** Griseofulvin may precipitate acute porphyria attacks

Ref. Metabolic Control and Disease, 8th edn, p 968;
     Oxford Textbook of Psychiatry, p 330

5.5 A **True** Calcification of the basal ganglia occurs
    B **True** Calcification of the basal ganglia occurs
    C **False** This is a rapidly growing cerebral tumour in which calcification does not develop
    D **True**
    E **True** The calcification tends to be patchy

Ref. Brain's Diseases of the Nervous System, 8th edn, pp 258–259,
     287–288, 662, 1140–1141

5.6 **All true**

Ref. British National Formulary, number 14, p 37

5.7 All true

Ref. Davidson's Principles and Practice of Medicine, 13th edn,
pp 715–716

5.8 A **False**
B **True**   This is the term for eating soil
C **False**
D **True**
E **True**

Ref. Oxford Textbook of Psychiatry, p 645;
Comprehensive Textbook of Psychiatry, 4th edn, p 1734

5.9 A **False**
B **False**
C **True**
D **True**
E **True**

Ref. Oxford Textbook of Psychiatry, pp 647–648

5.10 All false

Ref. Oxford Textbook of Psychiatry, p 650

5.11 A **True**
B **True**
C **True**
D **False**   Benzodiazepines may increase overactivity
E **False**

Ref. Oxford Textbook of Psychiatry, pp 657–659

5.12 A **True**
B **False**
C **False**
D **True**
E **True**

Ref. Oxford Textbook of Psychiatry, pp 660–662

5.13 A **False**
B **True**
C **True**
D **True**
E **True**

Ref. Oxford Textbook of Psychiatry, p 117

5.14 All true

Ref. Oxford Textbook of Psychiatry, pp 151–152

5.15 A **False**   It occurs more often in agoraphobia
    B **False**   They occur more often in agoraphobia
    C **False**   It occurs more often in agoraphobia
    D **True**
    E **False**   Like agoraphobics, patients with social phobic
                    neuroses think about the situation in advance and
                    often feel anxious long before encountering them

    Ref. Oxford Textbook of Psychiatry, p 159

5.16 A **False**   This is a conversion symptom
    B **True**
    C **False**   This is a conversion symptom
    D **True**
    E **True**

    Ref. Oxford Textbook of Psychiatry, p 170

5.17 All true

    Ref. Handbook of Affective Disorders, p 191;
          Oxford Textbook of Psychiatry, pp 325–329

5.18 A **True**   Schneiderian first-rank symptoms have been
                    reported in approximately 8–23% of manic patients
                    (Carpenter et al 1973; Taylor & Abrams 1973)
    B **True**
    C **True**
    D **True**
    E **False**   This is a particular form of severe depressive
                    disorder

    Ref. Handbook of Affective Disorders, p 15;
          Oxford Textbook of Psychiatry, pp 190, 192

5.19 A **False**
    B **True**
    C **True**
    D **False**
    E **True**

    Ref. Oxford Textbook of Psychiatry, p 261;
          Companion to Psychiatric Studies, 4th edn, p 325

5.20 A **True**   The average weight loss is approximately 5% by age
                    70, 10% by 80, 20% by 90
    B **False**   Ventricular enlargement occurs
    C **False**   The meninges thicken with age
    D **True**
    E **False**   There is a minor and selective loss

    Ref. Oxford Textbook of Psychiatry, p 493

5.21 All true

Ref. Oxford Textbook of Psychiatry, p 501

5.22 A **False**   This is a feature of the advanced stage
B **True**
C **True**
D **True**
E **True**

Ref. Oxford Textbook of Psychiatry, p 506;
Companion to Psychiatric Studies, 4th edn, p 280–281

5.23 All true

Ref. Oxford Textbook of Psychiatry, p 173;
Companion to Psychiatric Studies, 4th edn, p 367

5.24 All false

Ref. Handbook of Affective Disorders, p 279

5.25 A **False**   Paykel (1978) calculated that, in the 6 months after an event, the risks of illness are increased by between 2 and 7 times, depending on the severity of the event and the type of illness. The risks were least for schizophrenia out of the illnesses studied
B **True**   The risks were least for schizophrenia out of the illnesses studied
C **False**   Of the illnesses studied suicide attempts were found to have the greatest association with life events
D **True**   Of the illnesses studied suicide attempts were found to have the greatest association with life events
E **False**   The relative risk is a good measure of the magnitude of the causative effect of life event stress

Ref. Paykel E S 1978 Psychological Medicine 8: 245–253;
Andrews J G, Tennent C 1978 Psychological Medicine 8: 547;
Companion to Psychiatric Studies, 4th edn, p 379;
Oxford Textbook of Psychiatry, p 92

5.26 A **True**   Between 3.5 and 4.0 per 1000
B **False**   It changed little. The incidence fell, but patients lived longer, particularly those with Down's syndrome
C **False**   It fell by approximately one-third
D **False**   Tizard defined the administrative prevalence as the numbers for whom services would be required in a community which made provision for all who needed them. It falls after the age of 16, being greater in childhood
E **False**

Ref. Oxford Textbook of Psychiatry, pp 688–689

5.27 All true

> **Ref**. Oxford Textbook of Psychiatry, p 527;
> British National Formulary number 15, pp 83–84

5.28 A **True**
B **True**
C **True**
D **True**
E **False**   Prolongation, not shortening, of the QT interval is a recognized side-effect

> **Ref**. Oxford Textbook of Psychiatry, pp 544–545;
> British National Formulary number 15, p 153

5.29 A **False**
B **True**
C **False**   ECT has occassionally been administered to children (Frommer 1968; Hift et al 1960)
D **False**
E **True**

> **Ref**. Treatment and Management in Adult Psychiatry, p 131

5.30 A **True**
B **True**
C **True**
D **False**   Fregoli was an actor; Fregoli's illusion was named after him
E **True**

> **Ref**. Oxford Textbook of Psychiatry, pp 11–12

5.31 A **True**   Lima collaborated with Moniz in performing the first series of 20 psychosurgical operations in 1936
B **False**
C **True**   Together with Freeman, he modified Moniz's operation and devised the standard prefrontal leucotomy
D **True**   Lima collaborated with Moniz in performing the first series of 20 psychosurgical operations in 1936
E **False**   He is known for his work in psychotherapy

> **Ref**. Companion to Psychiatric Studies, 4th edn, pp 721–722;
> Treatment and Management in Adult Psychiatry, p 150

5.32 A **False** He has made important contributions to the study of deliberate self-harm and suicide
B **False** He has made important contributions to the study of group therapy
C **True**
D **True**
E **True**

Ref. Treatment and Management in Adult Psychiatry, chapter 25; Companion to Psychiatric Studies, 4th edn, chapter 30

5.33 A **False** 'Abnormal homicide'
B **True**
C **False** 'Abnormal homicide'
D **False** 'Abnormal homicide'
E **True**

Ref. Oxford Textbook of Psychiatry, p 731; Companion to Psychiatric Studies, 4th edn, p 673

5.34 A **False**
B **False**
C **True** The motive for fire-setting may be excitement or revenge on someone in authority (Reid 1982)
D **False**
E **True** The rate of detection is high since the exposer is often known to the victim

Ref. Oxford Textbook of Psychiatry, pp 722–723

5.35 All true

Ref. Oxford Textbook of Psychiatry, pp 737–738

5.36 A **False** According to Freud, this is one of the principles that governs mental activity
B **False** Associated with Carl G. Jung
C **True** This refers to the inability of the adolescent to accept the role he or she believes is expected by society
D **False** Associated with Sullivan
E **True** This refers to the stages of ego and social development

Ref. Comprehensive Textbook of Psychiatry, 4th edn, pp 371–373, 378, 427, 436

5.37 A **False** Written by J. D. Frank
B **False** Written by S. Freud
C **False** Written by S. Freud
D **False** Written by I. Yalom
E **False** Written by M. Balint

5.38 A **True**
       B **False**
       C **False**
       D **True**
       E **False**

Ref. Comprehensive Textbook of Psychiatry, 4th edn, pp 425–453

5.39 A **True**
       B **True**
       C **True**
       D **True**
       E **False**

Ref. Treatment and Management in Adult Psychiatry, p 181

5.40 A **True**
       B **True**
       C **False**
       D **True**
       E **True**

Ref. Fairburn R 1958 On the nature and aims of psycho-analytical
       treatment;
       Symington N 1986 The analytic experience. Free Association Books,
       London

A B   perinatal.
C, D   antenatal
E   post natal

5.41 All true

Ref. Oxford Textbook of Psychiatry, p 695

5.42 All true

Ref. Companion to Psychiatric Studies, 4th edn, pp 53, 484, 561;
       Oxford Textbook of Psychiatry, p 426

5.43 A **False**   William Gull described anorexia nervosa in 1868.
                 Russell described bulimia nervosa as an ominous
                 variant of anorexia nervosa in 1979
       B **False**   However, this condition is much more common in
                 females
       C **True**
       D **True**
       E **False**

Ref. Oxford Textbook of Psychiatry, p 370;
       Bulimia Nervosa — Current Approaches;
       Lacey J H, Dolan B M 1988 Bulimia in British Blacks and Asians.
       British Journal of Psychiatry 152: 73

5.44 A **False**   Schedule 2
B **False**   Schedule 3
C **True**
D **False**   Schedule 3
E **True**

Ref. British National Formulary, number 15, pp 8–9

5.45 A **False**
B **True**
· C **True**
D **False**
E **True**

Ref. British National Formulary, number 15, p 9

5.46 All true   Plumbism is lead poisoning

Ref. Comprehensive Textbook of Psychiatry, 4th edn, p 1083

5.47 A **False**   Rape is not usual following the act of exposure
B **False**   They seldom practise voyeurism
C **False**   Most choose places from which escape is easy
D **True**
E **False**   There is no satisfactory evidence about the value of group psychotherapy

Ref. Oxford Textbook of Psychiatry, pp 480–481

5.48 A **True**
B **True**
C **True**
D **False**
E **True**

Ref. Companion to Psychiatric Studies, 4th edn, chapter 39

5.49 A **True**
B **False**
C **True**
D **True**
E **True**

Ref. Companion to Psychiatric Studies, 4th edn, chapter 39

5.50 All true

Ref. Companion to Psychiatric Studies, 4th edn, chapter 39

PAPER 6: SHORT-ANSWER QUESTION PAPER

6.1 Numbness phase — Feeling of unreality. Lasts for a few hours
to 2 weeks
Main phase — Mourning. Sadness, weeping, poor sleep
anorexia, restlessness, irritability. Difficulty concentrating.
Occasionally, brief hallucinations. May last several weeks to
several months but with possible recurrences later, e.g. at
anniversaries that are reminders of the deceased
Acceptance phase — Readjustment at new situation. Several
weeks after the death
Differences
Suicidal thoughts far less frequent in bereavement than in
depressive disorders
Guilt about past actions in general much commoner in
depressive disorders compared with guilt about not doing
enough for the deceased in bereavement
In bereavement, more likely to complain of physical symptoms
Retardation uncommon after bereavement compared with
depressive disorders
(Give any three)

> **Ref.** Companion Psychiatric Studies, 3rd edn, pp 565–566;
> Oxford Textbook of Psychiatry, p 194

6.2 **Schneider's first-rank symptoms of schizophrenia** (in the
absence of organic disease)
Thought insertion
Thought withdrawal
Thought broadcasting
Somatic passivity
'Made' acts/drives/affect
Delusional perception
Auditory hallucinations
- audible thoughts
- voices arguing about subjects
- voices commenting on actions in the third person
Empirical research has shown that Schneider's first-rank
symptoms give little information about the prognosis of the
disease in a given patient

> **Ref.** Berrios G E 1987 Practical Reviews in Psychiatry, Series 2, 3, 7;
> Treatment and Management in Adult Psychiatry, pp 284–286

6.3   Commonest at three periods — between 5 and 7, at 11, and at 14 years and older. The second period may be associated with change of school
Mothers overprotective whilst fathers may be passive
Separation anxiety may be a cause, particularly in younger children
True phobia of school or of travel to and from school may be a cause in older children
Often 'model children' who have done well at school and have high standards
Other notes — classification, course, prognosis, etc.

> **Ref.** Companion to Psychiatric Studies, 4th edn, pp 523–524, 547;
> Oxford Textbook of Psychiatry, pp 650–651

6.4   The testator should be examined alone
Relatives and friends should be seen to check the accuracy of statements
The following legal criteria should be used when examining the testator:
   • whether the testator understands both the act of making a will and its consequences
   • whether the testator has a reasonable knowledge of the nature and extent of his or her property
   • whether the testator knows and appreciates the claims to which he or she ought to give effect
   • whether the testator is not influenced in making the will by any abnormal emotional state or delusions

> **Ref.** Oxford Textbook of Psychiatry, p 718;
> Companion to Psychiatric Studies, 4th edn. p 668

6.5   Projection
Denial
Rationalization
Introjection
Repression
Reaction formation
Magical undoing
Splitting
Sublimation
Displacement of affect, etc.

> **Ref.** Comprehensive Textbook of Psychiatry, 4th edn, pp 388–390;
> Oxford Textbook of Psychiatry, pp 30–31;
> Companion to Psychiatric Studies, 4th edn, p 76

6.6   Delirium tremens is a withdrawal symptom that may occur in chronic heavy drinkers and problem drinkers 2–4 days after the intake of alcohol has been stopped or reduced, although prodromal features may occur earlier. It is uncommon — 5% of alcoholics attending clinics have experienced it

Features

Clouding of consciousness, disorientation, and impairment of recent memory

Perceptual distortions — including vivid visual hallucinations

Agitation and restlessness

Tremor of hands, body and tongue

Insomnia

Autonomic disturbances — tachycardia, raised blood pressure, sweating, dilated pupils, etc.

Dehydration

Electrolyte disturbance

Hypokalaemia

Ref. Oxford Textbook of Psychiatry, p 427;
Companion to Psychiatric Studies, 4th edn, pp 262, 490;
Comprehensive Textbook of Psychiatry, 4th edn, p 1023

6.7   Depressive illness

Drug therapy — may need to use a tricyclic antidepressant with low cardiotoxicity, or another type of antidepressant, e.g. mianserin. Commence with minimum dose, usually as a single evening dose to improve sleep, reduce side-effects and improve compliance

Electroconvulsive therapy if:

● patient has failed to respond to medication
● risk of suicide
● poor food or fluid intake

Social and psychotherapeutic measures

Treat any underlying physical disease which may have precipitated the illness

Mania

General nursing care — note patient may be dehydrated and exhausted, hence fluid and food intake monitoring and encouragement important

Drug therapy

● e.g. haloperidol
● consider low-dose lithium carbonate prophylaxis

Ref. Treatment and Management in Adult Psychiatry, pp 455–456

6.8 **a.** Hyperthyroidism
  Phaeochromocytoma
  Hyperventilation
  Hypoglycaemia
  Drug withdrawal
  Neurological disorders, etc.
  (Give any five)
  b. Anaemia
  Sleep disorder
  Diabetes mellitus
  Infection
  Drug side-effects
  Addison's disease/hypoadrenalism
  Carcinoma, etc.
  (Give any five)

  Ref. Oxford Textbook of Psychiatry, pp 325–327, 343–344, 352

6.9 Both partners are treated together
  They are helped to communicate better about their sexual
  relationship
  Sexual attitudes are discussed and sexual information given
  Sexual intercourse is banned until the later stages
  In the next stage of sensate focus, mutual non-genital caressing
  is encouraged
  At the next stage mutual masturbation is allowed, but
  intercourse continues to be banned
  Later, intercourse is allowed, with appropriate techniques being
  used for specific problems, e.g. the squeeze technique (or the
  stop–start method) for premature ejaculation; finger
  exploration of the vagina or the use of gradual dilators for
  vaginismus

  Ref. Oxford Textbook of Psychiatry, pp 465–466

6.10 Autonomic — dizziness, salivation, flushing, tachycardia
  Perceptual — hallucinations (visual, auditory, olfactory,
  gustatory, somatic); déjà vu
  Cognitive disturbances
  Affective — anxiety, fear
  Psychomotor — automatisms

  Ref. Companion to Psychiatric Studies, 4th edn, pp 299–300;
  Oxford Textbook of Psychiatry, p 335

6.11   **a.** The null hypothesis is the position that in an experimental procedure or otherwise, it is assumed that there is no difference between the experimental group(s) and the control. Any such differences that are found to exist are assumed to arise by chance (until proven otherwise)

       b. This is the error of rejecting the null hypothesis when the latter is true

       c. This is the error of accepting a false null hypothesis

       d. This is the probability of rejecting the null hypothesis when it is false

     Ref. The Scientific Basis of Psychiatry, pp 165, 167–169;
         Companion to Psychiatric Studies, 2nd edn, p 221

6.12   **a.** (i) In approximately 95% of cases, non-dysjunction during meiosis leads to trisomy 21, Down's syndrome
         (ii) In approximately 5% of cases, Down's syndrome results from the translocation of the long arm of a chromosome (13, 14, 15, 21 or 22)

       b. Oblique palpebral fissures
         Small flattened skull
         Single transverse palmar crease
         Tongue fissured
         Squint common
         Congenital cardiac pathology — 50%
         Mental retardation
         Often cheerful when younger, etc.

     Ref. Comprehensive Textbook of Psychiatry, 4th edn, pp 29–30;
         Companion to Psychiatric Studies, 4th edn, pp 57, 194, 441–442

6.13   The dopamine hypothesis of schizophrenia postulates that certain dopaminergic pathways, often thought to be the mesolimbic-cortical bundles, are overactive in schizophrenia

Supportive evidence

- Drugs such as L-dopa and amphetamine potentiate dopaminergic activity, and can induce or exacerbate schizophrenic symptoms
- Symptoms of schizophrenia are relieved by neuroleptic drugs which are dopamine receptor antagonists
- Disulfiram may exacerbate schizophrenia, and is known to inhibit the conversion of dopamine to noradrenaline, by blocking the enzyme dopamine-β-hydroxylase
- Some studies of post-mortem brains in schizophrenia indicate increased dopamine receptors in certain parts (although there is the possibility that this is secondary to neuroleptic administration)
- Mescaline is an ortho-methylated derivative of dopamine, and is a known hallucinogen. Therefore some feel that perhaps the brain produces hallucinogens in schizophrenia

     Ref. Oxford Textbook of Psychiatry, p 258;
         Companion to Psychiatric Studies, 4th edn, pp 119, 321

6.14 Hippocampal formation — hippocampus, dentate gyrus, parahippocampal gyrus
Amygdaloid nucleus
Limbic lobe — cingulate gyrus, subcallosal gyrus, parahippocampal gyrus
Thalamus — anterior nucleus
Hypothalamus
(Note that textbooks differ in how broadly the limbic system is defined)
Normal functions
Sexual activity
Conditioned reflexes
Recent memory
Aggressive behaviour, anger, fear
(Give any three)

> **Ref.** Companion to Psychiatric Studies, 4th edn, pp 98–101;
> Clinical Neuroanatomy for Medical Students, 2nd edn,
> pp 309–315

6.15 Dysarthria is the imperfect articulation of speech.
Causes
Mechanical causes, e.g. ill-fitting dentures, cleft-palate
Stutter
Paralysis of any of cranial nerves VII, IX, X or XII
Parkinson's disease
Cerebellar disease
Pseudobulbar palsy
Progressive bulbar palsy
General paralysis of the insane
(Give any six)

> **Ref.** Davidson's Principles and Practice of Medicine, 13th edn, p 661;
> Comprehensive Textbook of Psychiatry, 4th edn, pp 86, 150;
> Lecture Notes on Clinical Medicine, 2nd edn, p 12

6.16 Based on statistical analysis of large numbers of subjects' responses. Identified three independent variables to describe personality
  (i) introversion–extraversion
  (ii) neuroticism–stability
  (iii) psychoticism
Postulates that score on scale (i) depends on functioning of the reticular activating system; score on (ii) depends on variation in the reactivity of the autonomic nervous system
Introverts are said to be more easily conditioned and develop stronger extinction-resistant responses than extraverts
High neuroticism — more likely to develop neurotic symptoms under stress

> **Ref.** The Scientific Basis of Psychiatry, pp 370–372;
> Companion to Psychiatric Studies, 4th edn, pp 45–46, 408–409

6.17 **a.** Fine tremor
Gastrointestinal disturbances — nausea, vomiting, diarrhoea
Urinary frequency
Polydipsia
Weight gain
Oedema
Muscle weakness, etc.
(Give any five)
  b. Drowsiness
Coarse tremor
Slurred speech
Ataxia
Confusion
Blurred vision
Hyper-reflexia and hyperextension of limbs
Convulsions, etc.
(Give any five)
  c. Nephrogenic diabetes insipidus
Tardive dyskinesia
Cardiotoxicity
Hypokalaemia
Exacerbation of psoriasis
Hypothyroidism, etc.
(Give any five)

Ref. Treatment and Management in Adult Psychiatry, pp 78–82;
British National Formulary, number 15, p 151

6.18 Matching — prospective, e.g. of sex or age
Randomization
Double-blind procedure — during the trial both the subject and
the experimenter are kept unaware of which treatment the
subject is receiving
Use of placebos — to measure the placebo response
Choosing an appropriate treatment regime
Choosing appropriate rating scales and measuring instruments
— a rating scale should not simply be chosen because it is
commonly used

Ref. The Scientific Basis of Psychiatry, pp 170–172

6.19   **a.** Raphe complex
Locus coeruleus
Gigantocellular tegmental field
(Give any two)

b. Dreaming
Increased pulse
Increased blood pressure
Increased respiration rate
Intermittent bursts of jerky rapid eye movements
Abolition of muscle tone in most skeletal muscles
Loss of most stretch reflexes
Penile erection or increased vaginal blood flow
EEG resembles that of full consciousness

Ref. Treatment and Management in Adult Psychiatry, pp 460–463;
Comprehensive Textbook of Psychiatry, 4th edn, pp 57–61;
Companion to Psychiatric Studies, 3rd edn, pp 177–178

6.20   **Oral stage** — 0–1 year old (approximately) — Pleasure from
sucking and other oral activities
Anal stage — 1–2 years old (approximately) — Divided into
anal-expulsive and anal-retentive. Activity centres around faecal
expulsion and faecal retention
Phallic stage — 3–5 years old (approximately) — Includes
urethral eroticism and oedipal–Electra complex
Latency stage — 5–12 years old (approximately) — Little
psychosexual development
Genital stage — 12–adulthood — Subject reaches full
heterosexual development

Ref. Comprehensive Textbook of Psychiatry, 4th edn, pp 359–362;
Oxford Textbook of Psychiatry, p 102

PAPER 7: MULTIPLE CHOICE QUESTIONS ON BASIC SCIENCES

7.1   A **False**   Infants begin to show selective smiling at between 3
and 5 months
B **False**
C **False**
D **True**
E **True**

Ref. Companion to Psychiatric Studies, 4th edn, pp 67–68

7.2   A **True**
B **True**
C **False**
D **False**
E **True**   Harlow & Griffin (1965)

Ref. The Scientific Basis of Psychiatry, pp 435–437

7.3 A **False**
  B **False**
  C **True**
  D **True**
  E **True**

Ref. Companion to Psychiatric Studies, 4th edn, p 520;
  The Scientific Principles of Psychopathology, chapter 9

7.4 A **True**
  B **True**
  C **False**
  D **True**
  E **True**

Ref. Companion to Psychiatric Studies, 4th edn, p 74;
  Comprehensive Textbook of Psychiatry, 4th edn, pp 1599–1600

7.5 A **False**   It was described by Festinger
  B **True**
  C **True**
  D **False**
  E **True**

Ref. Introduction to Psychology, 8th edn, pp 548–549

7.6 A **False**   This is the Wechsler Intelligence Scale for Children
  B **True**
  C **True**
  D **False**   This is the Wechsler Adult Intelligence Scale
  E **True**

Ref. Companion to Psychiatric Studies, 4th edn, pp 408–409;
  Introduction to Psychology, 8th edn, p 409

7.7 A **True**
  B **False**   This is seen in parietal lobe dysfunction
  C **True**
  D **False**
  E **True**

Ref. Companion to Psychiatric Studies, 4th edn, pp 258–260;
  Oxford Textbook of Psychiatry, pp 302–303

7.8 A **False**
  B **True**
  C **False**   It occurs in dominant parietal lobe lesions
  D **False**
  E **True**

Ref. Companion to Psychiatric Studies, 4th edn, p 261

7.9 A **False**   The acetylcholine action is described as muscarinic at these sites — the drug muscarine is an agonist at these receptors; however, the transmitter is acetylcholine

B **False**
C **False**
D **False**
E **False**   It is the sympathetic (not parasympathetic) supply

Ref. Companion to Psychiatric Studies, 4th edn, p 96

7.10 A **False**
B **True**   DOPA is 3,4-dihydroxyphenylalanine
C **True**
D **False**
E **False**

Ref. Companion to Psychiatric Studies, 4th edn, p 118

7.11 A **True**
B **True**
C **False**   GABA is an inhibitory central neurotransmitter
D **True**
E **True**   Somatostatin is excitatory in some parts of the brain

Ref. Companion to Psychiatric Studies, 4th edn, chapter 7

7.12 A **False**
B **True**
C **False**
D **False**
E **True**

Ref. Clinical Neuroanatomy for Medical Students, 2nd edn, pp 449–450

7.13 A **True**
B **False**
C **True**
D **True**
E **True**

Ref. Companion to Psychiatric Studies, 4th edn, pp 98–101;
Clinical Neuroanatomy for Medical Students, 2nd edn, pp 309–311

7.14 A **False**
B **True**
C **True**
D **True**
E **True**

Ref. Lecture Notes on Clinical Medicine, 2nd edn, p 8

7.15 A **True**
B **False**   This is a diencephalic structure
C **False**   These are mesencephalic structures
D **True**
E **False**   These are telencephalic structures

Ref. Companion to Psychiatric Studies, 4th edn, p 87

7.16 A **True**   From 5-HT
B **True**   From dopamine
C **True**   From histamine
D **True**   From noradrenaline
E **False**   This is a neurotransmitter

Ref. Companion to Psychiatric Studies, 4th edn, chapter 7

7.17 A **True**
B **True**
C **False**
D **True**
E **False**

Ref. Companion to Psychiatric Studies, 4th edn, chapter 7

7.18 A **True**
B **False**   Opioid kappa receptors are probably involved in this
C **True**
D **False**   Opioid sigma receptors are probably involved in this
E **True**

Ref. Companion to Psychiatric Studies, 3rd edn, p 145

7.19 A **True**
B **True**
C **False**   Chlorpromazine is a dopamine antagonist, and dopamine is prolactin inhibitory factor
D **False**   It has weak anticholinergic activity
E **True**

Ref. The Scientific Basis of Psychiatry, chapter 13

7.20 A **True**
B **False**
C **True**
D **True**
E **True**

Ref. The Scientific Basis of Psychiatry, chapter 13; British National Formulary, number 15, pp 143–146

7.21 All true

Ref. The Scientific Basis of Psychiatry, p 180; British National Formulary, number 15, pp 135–139

7.22 A **False**
B **True**
C **False**   Cocaine causes this
D **False**   Tetrahydro-cannabinol
E **True**

Ref. British National Formulary, number 15, p 7;
Oxford Textbook of Psychiatry, pp 450–451;
Companion to Psychiatric Studies, 4th edn, pp 487

7.23 A **False**   Tachycardia is a side-effect
B **False**
C **True**
D **True**
E **False**   Constipation is a side-effect

Ref. British National Formulary, number 15, p 153

7.24 A **True**
B **False**   They reduce REM sleep
C **True**
D **True**
E **True**

Ref. British National Formulary, number 15, pp 156–158;
The Scientific Basis of Psychiatry, pp 194–197

7.25 A **True**
B **False**
C **True**
D **False**
E **True**

Ref. Companion to Psychiatric Studies, 4th edn, pp 15–16

7.26 A **False**   It was first used by Main
B **True**
C **True**
D **True**
E **False**

Ref. Companion to Psychiatric Studies, 4th edn, pp 18–19

7.27 A **False**
B **True**
C **True**
D **True**
E **True**

Ref. Companion to Psychiatric Studies, 3rd edn, pp 25–26;
Oxford Textbook of Psychiatry, p 175

7.28 All true

Ref. Companion to Psychiatric Studies, 4th edn, p 21

7.29 All true

Ref. Basic Sociology, 4th edn, p 70

7.30 A **True**
B **True**
C **True**
D **True**
E **True**   Brown & Harris found that lower social class was a vulnerability factor; however, all the effect due to it was explained by the other four factors

Ref. Handbook of Affective Disorders, pp 118–119; Oxford Textbook of Psychiatry, pp 206–207; Companion to Psychiatric Studies, 4th edn, p 350

7.31 A **True**
B **False**
C **False**   They are chromatin-positive
D **True**
E **True**

Ref. Companion to Psychiatric Studies, 4th edn, pp 161, 185, 443

7.32 A **True**
B **True**
C **True**
D **False**
E **True**

Ref. The Scientific Basis of Psychiatry, chapter 16; Companion to Psychiatric Studies, 3rd edn, chapter 9

7.33 A **True**
B **False**
C **False**
D **True**   This is tuberous sclerosis
E **True**

Ref. The Scientific Basis of Psychiatry, chapter 16; Companion to Psychiatric Studies, 3rd edn, chapter 9

7.34 A **False**
B **True**   Trisomy 21
C **True**   Trisomy 13
D **False**
E **True**   Trisomy 18

Ref. The Scientific Basis of Psychiatry, chapter 16; Companion to Psychiatric Studies, 4th edn, chapter 9

7.35 A **False**
B **True**
C **False**   Environmental factors are also involved
D **True**
E **True**

Ref. The Scientific Basis of Psychiatry, chapter 14;
Companion to Psychiatric Studies, 4th edn, chapter 9

7.36 A **False**   This is a disorder of amino acid metabolism
B **True**
C **True**
D **True**
E **False**   This is a disorder of amino acid metabolism

Ref. Companion to Psychiatric Studies, 4th edn, pp 147–150;
Oxford Textbook of Psychiatry, pp 695–696

7.37 A **True**   Sex-linked disorders that usually only occur in males
may occur in Turner's syndrome because there is
only one X chromosome

B **True**
C **True**
D **False**   Very occasionally down-growths of germinal
epithelium may occur in the ovaries, and sometimes
even primordial follicles. This may account for the
very rare cases of menstrual bleeding in this
condition

E **True**

Ref. The Scientific Basis of Psychiatry, pp 253–257

7.38 **All true**   Mental retardation is present continuously from early
life and personality disorder continuously from the
end of adolescence, whilst mental illness is said to
have a recognizable onset following normal
functioning in adult life

Ref. Oxford Textbook of Psychiatry, pp 69–70

7.39 A **True**
B **True**
C **False**
D **True**
E **True**

Ref. Oxford Textbook of Psychiatry, p 229

7.40 A **True**
   B **False**   This is a DSM-III R classification
   C **False**   This is a DSM-III R classification
   D **False**   This is a DSM-III R classification
   E **True**

   Ref. Oxford Textbook of Psychiatry, pp 133–135

7.41 A **False**
   B **False**
   C **True**
   D **True**
   E **True**

   Ref. Oxford Textbook of Psychiatry, pp 400–401

7.42 All true

   Ref. Oxford Textbook of Psychiatry, p 433

7.43 A **False**   The median is always equal to the mode
   B **True**
   C **False**   The mean is always equal to the mode
   D **False**   The proportion is approximately 68%
   E **False**   The proportion is approximately 95%

   Ref. Companion to Psychiatric Studies, 2nd edn, p 218

7.44 A **False**
   B **False**
   C **False**
   D **True**
   E **False**

   Ref. Companion to Psychiatric Studies, 2nd edn, chapter 14

7.45 A **True**   Mean $= \Sigma x/n$
   B **False**   The required interval is given by [(mean $- 2s$) to (mean $+ 2s$)], where s is the standard error of the mean. Now, the mean $= 90$ (given), and $s = 3$ (see part C of this question). Therefore the interval is [(90 $- 6$) to (90 $+ 6$)], i.e. [84 to 96]
   C **True** $s =$ (standard deviation)/(square root of n), where n is the sample size. Thus $s = 12/4 = 3$
   D **False**   It is more appropriate to use the t-distribution because n is less than 30
   E **True**   Variance $=$ standard deviation squared $= 12 \times 12 = 144$

   Ref. Companion to Psychiatric Studies, 2nd edn, chapter 14

7.46 A **True**
B **True**
C **True**
D **False**   Unless it is a cross-over trial
E **False**   Unless it is a cross-over trial

Ref. Companion to Psychiatric Studies, 2nd edn, p 232;
Companion to Psychiatric Studies, 3rd edn, pp 604–605

7.47 **All true**   The placebo effect is a measure of the psychological effects of the effect of being treated, as opposed to a measure of the response of subjects who have had no treatment at all. The Hawthorne effect is the better response that may occur from subjects who believe that an interest is being taken in them

Ref. Companion to Psychiatric Studies, 2nd edn, p 232;
The Scientific Basis of Psychiatry, pp 171–172

7.48 A **False**   A correlation coefficient of zero implies complete absence of correlation
B **True**
C **False**   This would be the case when the correlation coefficient is less than zero
D **True**
E **False**

Ref. Statistics at Square One, chapter 11

7.49 A **True**
B **True**
C **True**
D **False**   Chi-squared $= \Sigma[(fo - fe)/fe]$. But the value of the number of degrees of freedom is needed to calculate the value of p
E **True**   See the answer to D above

Ref. Companion to Psychiatric Studies, 2nd edn, chapter 14;
Statistics at Square One, chapter 8

7.50 A **True**
B **False**
C **True**
D **True**
E **True**

Ref. Companion to Psychiatric Studies, 2nd edn, chapter 14.

PAPER 8: MULTIPLE CHOICE QUESTIONS ON CLINICAL TOPICS

8.1 **All true** These were proposed by Karl Bonhoeffer, who was Professor of Psychiatry in Berlin

Ref. Oxford Textbook of Psychiatry, p 295

8.2 A **True** It has been used for the involuntary movements but there is a risk of worsening the dementia or causing neurological side-effects

B **True**
C **False** It is most marked in the frontal lobes
D **True**
E **False** Cases have been reported at the two extremes of life

Ref. Oxford Textbook of Psychiatry, pp 312–313;
Companion to Psychiatric Studies, 4th edn, pp 288–289

8.3 A **False** Volunteers who smoked the drug at a dose of 0.2 mg/kg did show some short-term psychotic reactions. However, there is no convincing evidence for more prolonged psychotic disturbances — although some cases have been reported, it has never been fully established that such patients had not suffered from some pre-existing psychotic tendency (Edwards 1976)

B **True**
C **True**
D **True**
E **True**

Ref. Oxford Textbook of Psychiatry, pp 240–241, 451;
Companion to Psychiatric Studies, 4th edn, p 487

8.4 A **False** It is the time between the head injury and the resumption of normal continuous memory

B **False** Post-traumatic amnesia lasting 1–24 h was defined as moderate concussion by Russell & Smith (1961)

C **False** Post-traumatic amnesia lasting 1–7 days was defined as severe concussion by Russell & Smith (1961). Post-traumatic amnesia lasting more than 7 days was defined as very severe concussion

D **True**
E **True**

Ref. Oxford Textbook of Psychiatry, p 315;
Companion to Psychiatric Studies, 3rd edn, pp 265–266

8.5 A **True**
  B **False**   The prothrombin time is prolonged
  C **False**   Hyperventilation occurs in association with hepatic
           failure
  D **False**   Hepatic failure usually develops after 4 days
  E **False**

Ref. British National Formulary, number 15, p 38

8.6 A **True**
  B **False**   It causes hypotension
  C **True**
  D **False**
  E **True**

Ref. Companion to Psychiatric Studies, 4th edn, p 267;
     Oxford Textbook of Psychiatry, p 326

8.7 A **False**   It may confirm, but it cannot exclude this diagnosis
  B **True**
  C **True**
  D **True**
  E **True**

Ref. Oxford Textbook of Psychiatry, pp 306, 337

8.8 A **True**
  B **False**
  C **True**
  D **True**
  E **False**   Lack of drive occurs

Ref. Oxford Textbook of Psychiatry, p 318

8.9 A **False**   It occurs in child abuse
  B **True**
  C **True**
  D **False**
  E **True**

Ref. Oxford Textbook of Psychiatry, pp 646–647

8.10 A **True**
  B **False**   This is a common childhood ritual
  C **False**   This is a common childhood ritual
  D **True**   The child may ask its parents to take part in rituals or
           to give repeated reassurances about obsessional
           thoughts
  E **True**

Ref. Oxford Textbook of Psychiatry, pp 648–649;
     Companion to Psychiatric Studies, 4th edn, p 523

8.11 A **True**
   B **True**
   C **False**
   D **False**   Juvenile delinquency is not a psychiatric diagnosis but a legal category
   E **False**   Genetic factors appear to be of only minor importance in the aetiology of delinquency (Shields 1980)

Ref.   Oxford Textbook of Psychiatry, pp 654–655

8.12 A **True**
   B **False**   It was first described by Kanner (1943)
   C **False**   The prevalence is approximately 20 per 100 000 children
   D **False**   It is more frequent in the upper socioeconomic classes
   E **True**

Ref.   Oxford Textbook of Psychiatry, pp 659–661

8.13 A **True**   301.0
   B **False**   This is a DSM-III R category — 301.81
   C **False**   This is a DSM-III R category — 301.83
   D **False**   This is a DSM-III R category — 301.84
   E **True**   301.6

Ref.   Mental Disorders: Glossary and Guide to their Classification in Accordance with the Ninth Revision of the International Classification of Diseases;
Diagnostic and Statistical Manual of Mental Disorders, 3rd edn — revised;
Oxford Textbook of Psychiatry, p 110

8.14 A **True**
   B **True**
   C **False**
   D **True**
   E **True**   This is the same as leptosomatic

Ref.   Oxford Textbook of Psychiatry, p 119

8.15 A **True**
   B **True**
   C **True**   Because of aerophagy
   D **False**   Failure of erection and loss of libido are common
   E **True**

Ref.   Oxford Textbook of Psychiatry, pp 150–151

8.16 A **True**
  B **True**
  C **False**   Depersonalization may be a dissociative symptom
  D **False**   This is a dissociative symptom
  E **True**

  Ref. Oxford Textbook of Psychiatry, p 170;
      Companion to Psychiatric Studies, 4th edn, chapter 19

8.17 All true

  Ref. Handbook of Affective Disorders, pp 4, 6–7;
      Oxford Textbook of Psychiatry, pp 188–189

8.18 A **False**   It is commoner in males
  B **True**
  C **True**
  D **True**
  E **True**

  Ref. Treatment and Management in Adult Psychiatry, p 472

8.19 All false

  Ref. Oxford Textbook of Psychiatry, p 237;
      Companion to Psychiatric Studies, 4th edn, p 312

8.20 A **True**
  B **True**
  C **True**
  D **False**
  E **True**

  Ref. Oxford Textbook of Psychiatry, p 261;
      Companion to Psychiatric Studies, 4th edn, pp 324–326

8.21 A **True**
  B **False**
  C **False**
  D **True**
  E **False**

  Ref. Oxford Textbook of Psychiatry, p 495

8.22 A **False**   Impairment of consciousness is invariable —
          although it is not always obvious (e.g. when the
          onset is gradual)
  B **True**
  C **True**
  D **False**   Mortality is high because many of the causes of
          acute organic syndrome are a threat to life
  E **False**   Benzodiazepines may increase confusion

  Ref. Oxford Textbook of Psychiatry, p 504

8.23 A **True**
  B **True**
  C **True**
  D **True**
  E **False**

Ref. Handbook of Affective Disorders, pp 113–114, 117;
  Weissman M M, Klerman G L 1977 Sex differences and the
  epidemiology of depression. Archives of General Psychiatry
  34: 98–110

8.24 A **False** Systemic lupus erythematosus is not a common
          cause of presenile dementia
  B **False** Alzheimer's disease is the commonest cause of
          presenile dementia
  C **False** The correct prevalence is 4–7 per 100 000
  D **False** The female to male ratio is approximately 2 to 1
  E **False** In Huntington's chorea there is an equal sex ratio

Ref. Oxford Textbook of Psychiatry, pp 311–312, 324;
  Davidson's Principles and Practice of Medicine, 13th edn,
  pp 627–629

8.25 A **True**
  B **False**
  C **False** It has increased greatly
  D **True**   This was demonstrated by Plant (1979)
  E **True**

Ref. Oxford Textbook of Psychiatry, pp 431–433;
  Companion to Psychiatric Studies, 4th edn, pp 478–481

8.26 **All true** The prevalence was found to increase as intelligence
          decreased. A strong association was found between
          conduct disorder and reading retardation

Ref. Oxford Textbook of Psychiatry, p 631

8.27 A **True**   Causes sedation in the infant
  B **True**   The milk concentration may exceed maternal plasma
          concentrations fourfold and may lead to drowsiness
          in the infant
  C **False** This is present in the milk in amounts too small to be
          harmful
  D **False** This is present in the milk in amounts too small to be
          harmful
  E **False** This is present in the milk in amounts too small to be
          harmful

Ref. British National Formulary, number 15, pp 30–33

8.28 A **True**
    B **False**   It slows initially
    C **False**
    D **True**   Cerebral blood flow increases by up to 200%
    E **True**

    Ref. Oxford Textbook of Psychiatry, p 565;
          Treatment and Management in Adult Psychiatry, pp 139–140

8.29 A **True**
    B **False**
    C **True**
    D **False**
    E **True**

    Ref. British National Formulary, number 15, pp 75, 91–92, 213

8.30 All true

    Ref. Treatment and Management in Adult Psychiatry, chapter 21;
          Bulimia Nervosa — Current Approaches

8.31 A **False**   Alfred Adler is best known for his work in individual
                    psychology and psychotherapy
    B **True**
    C **True**
    D **True**
    E **True**

    Ref. Companion to Psychiatric Studies, 4th edn, chapter 27;
          Treatment and Management in Adult Psychiatry, chapter 24

8.32 A **True**
    B **True**
    C **False**   Janssen synthesized haloperidol. Kuhn described the
                    antidepressant effect of imipramine
    D **True**
    E **False**   Sternbach described the sedating effects of
                    chlordiazepoxide in 1957. Janssen synthesized
                    haloperidol

    Ref. Companion to Psychiatric Studies, 4th edn, p 682

8.33 A **False**   Female
    B **True**
    C **False**   They are likely to have had fewer previous
                    convictions than convicted homicide offenders
    D **True**
    E **True**

    Ref. Oxford Textbook of Psychiatry, p 732

8.34 A **False**   It cannot be decided in a magistrates' court
      B **True**
      C **True**
      D **True**
      E **True**

Ref. Companion to Psychiatric Studies, 4th edn, p 676;
        Oxford Textbook of Psychiatry, p 725

8.35 A **False**   Written by Carl G. Jung
      B **False**   Written by Carl G. Jung
      C **True**
      D **True**
      E **False**   Written by Anna Freud

8.36 A **True**   Also known as self-dynamism
      B **True**
      C **False**   Associated with Melanie Klein
      D **True**
      E **False**

Ref. Comprehensive Textbook of Psychiatry, 4th edn, pp 428–429, 443,
        471

8.37 A **False**   This was described by Alfred Adler
      B **True**
      C **False**   This is not a complex
      D **True**
      E **True**

Ref. Comprehensive Textbook of Psychiatry, 4th edn, pp 435–436

8.38 **All true**

Ref. Comprehensive Textbook of Psychiatry, 4th edn, pp 422–443

8.39 A **True**
      B **False**   Associated with Sigmund Freud
      C **True**
      D **True**
      E **True**

Ref. Comprehensive Textbook of Psychiatry, 4th edn, pp 455–456

8.40 A **True**
      B **False**   According to Freud, this is primary gain
      C **True**
      D **True**
      E **True**

Ref. Comprehensive Textbook of Psychiatry, 4th edn, p 920

8.41 A **True**
      B **True**
      C **True**
      D **True**
      E **False**   The overall IQ distribution of females with Turner's syndrome is near normal (although mean scores on arithmetical and visuospatial tasks are usually lower than those of normal female controls)

Ref. Oxford Textbook of Psychiatry, pp 695–696, 701;
       Companion to Psychiatric Studies, 4th edn, p 185

8.42 A **True**
      B **False**
      C **False**   It is more common in the upper than the lower social classes
      D **False**   It is usually normal, although the T_3 level may be reduced
      E **True**

Ref. Oxford Textbook of Psychiatry, pp 365–366

8.43 A **True**   This syndrome is caused by widespread demyelination of the optic tracts, cerebellar peduncles and corpus callosum
      B **True**
      C **False**
      D **True**
      E **True**

Ref. Oxford Textbook of Psychiatry, p 425

8.44 A **False**   This is related to the amphetamines and is a class C drug
      B **False**   This is related to the amphetamines and is a class C drug
      C **False**   A class A drug
      D **True**
      E **False**   A class C drug

Ref. British National Formulary, number 15, p 8

8.45 A **True**
      B **True**
      C **True**
      D **False**   It is less sedating than morphine
      E **False**   It is a class A drug

Ref. British National Formulary, number 15, pp 8, 171;
       Oxford Textbook of Psychiatry, p 447

8.46 A **True**
B **False**
C **True**
D **False**
E **True**

Ref. Comprehensive Textbook of Psychiatry, 4th edn, p 1084

8.47 A **False**   It occurs in 1 in 500 to 1 in 1000 births
B **True**
C **False**   The symptoms of maternity blues peak on the third or fourth postpartum day
D **True**   80% of cases were found to be affective by Dean & Kendell (1981)
E **True**   Most patients recover fully from a puerperal psychosis

Ref. Oxford Textbook of Psychiatry, pp 390–392

8.48 A **True**
B **True**   Although it was advocated primarily for the treatment of premature ejaculation, it can be helpful for erectile impotence if an erection has been produced by the 'genital focus' exercises of Masters & Johnson
C **False**   These are involved in some of the techniques of Masters & Johnson
D **True**
E **True**

Ref. Comprehensive Textbook of Psychiatry, 4th edn, p 1088; Treatment and Management in Adult Psychiatry, p 425

8.49 A **True**
B **True**
C **False**   This is a type of aversion therapy
D **False**
E **True**

Ref. Companion to Psychiatric Studies, 4th edn, chapter 39

8.50 A **False**
B **True**
C **True**
D **False**   This was described by Karen Horney
E **True**

Ref. Companion to Psychiatric Studies, 4th edn, p 775

PAPER 9: SHORT-ANSWER QUESTION PAPER

9.1   Schizophrenia
Illicit drug abuse — particularly amphetamines
Bipolar affective disorder
Temporal lobe epilepsy
The patient has invented the symptoms — this must always be
borne in mind with patients who are doctors or nurses
(particularly with this number of first-rank symptoms)
Iatrogenic, e.g. steroid psychosis, L-dopa
Hysteria
Personality disorder
(Give any five)

Ref. Oxford Textbook of Psychiatry, pp 245–246

9.2   Chronic subdural haematoma
Poorly controlled epileptic seizures
Liver disorder
Hypothyroidism
Normal pressure hydrocephalus
Anaemia
Congestive cardiac failure
Chronic pulmonary disease
Vitamin deficiency — including thiamine, nicotinic acid, vitamin
B_{12} and folic acid
Cerebral tumours

Ref. Treatment and Management in Adult Psychiatry, p 447

9.3   **Fetishism** — inanimate objects are the preferred or exclusive
method of achieving sexual excitement. Most are heterosexual.
Objects include clothes, e.g. female underclothes and rubber
clothes. Contact with the preferred object(s) may be followed by
intercourse with a partner wearing the fetish or by masturbation
Transvestism — male transvestism involves repeated dressing
in female clothes. Cross-dressing may start at puberty.
Transvestists experience erections when cross-dressing and
may masturbate. Most are heterosexual
Paedophilia — prepubertal children, in reality or in fantasy, are
the preferred or exclusive method of achieving sexual
excitement. Almost exclusively a male disorder. The child may
be male or female. Fondling and/or masturbation is commoner
than coitus with younger children, although cases of forcible
penetration do occur
Bestiality — animals are the preferred or exclusive method of
achieving sexual excitement. Also know as zoophilia or
bestiosexuality. Rarer than the above
Necrophilia — sexual arousal is achieved via coitus with a dead
body. The body may be that of a murdered victim, the murderer
then having intercourse with this body. Rarer than the above

Ref. Oxford Textbook of Psychiatry, pp 474–479

9.4 Depressive symptoms
Reversion to immature behaviour patterns
Increased anxiety
Destructive acts
Paranoid ideas
Complaints of somatic disorders
Guilt
Worsening of phobias
(Other include: generalization of existing phobias, hostility,
lowered self-esteem, loss of impulse control and suicide)

Ref. Treatment and Management in Adult Psychiatry, p 173

9.5 Depression
Anxiety
Excess caffeine
Excess alcohol
Dyspnoea
Pruritus, etc.

Ref. Oxford Textbook of Psychiatry, p 532

9.6 a. Previous episode(s) of violence
Repeated impulsive behaviour
Difficulty in coping with stress
Previous unwillingness to delay gratification
Sadistic traits
Paranoid traits
b. Morbid jealousy
Paranoid belief and a wish to harm others
Deceptiveness
Lack of self control
Threats of violence
Attitude to treatment

Ref. Oxford Textbook of Psychiatry, pp 742–743

9.7 Headache
Short-term amnesia
Temporary confusion
Small electrical burns
Muscle pain
Temporary nausea and vertigo
(Give any five)

Ref. Oxford Textbook of Psychiatry, p 566

9.8   Irrational fear of a specific object, activity or situation. Fear is irrational in the sense that it out of proportion to the real situation. Sufferer is aware that his or her reactions are irrational. Persistent avoidance behaviour occurs secondary to the above. Not under voluntary control

Treatment methods

Behaviour therapies — systematic desensitization, flooding (in vivo or in imagination), modelling;

Psychotropic medication

- benzodiazepines or β-adrenoceptor antagonists in combination with behaviour therapy
- tricyclic antidepressants
- monoamine oxidase inhibitors

Supportive psychotherapy

Psychodynamic psychotherapy

Ref. Comprehensive Textbook of Psychiatry, 4th edn, pp 895, 903–904

9.9   The defendant must be able to:

- understand the nature of the charge and its consequences
- understand the difference between pleading guilty and not guilty
- instruct counsel for the defence
- challenge the jurors
- follow the evidence presented in court

Ref. Oxford Textbook of Psychiatry, p 725;
     Companion to Psychiatric Studies, 4th edn, p 676

9.10   i. **Phenylketonuria** — detectable by postnatal screening of blood or urine. Excess phenylalanine in the blood — Guthrie test, or phenylpyruvic acid in the urine. Molecular genetic techniques can be applied using cloned DNA probes for the gene for phenylalanine hydroxylase. Treated by exclusion of phenylalanine from the diet

ii. **Galactosaemia** — detectable by postnatal screening of blood for lack of galactose-1-phosphate uridyl transferase. Treated by galactose-free diet

iii. **Cretinism** (hypothyroidism) — detectable by postnatal screening of blood for thyroid function tests. Treated with thyroxine

Ref. Oxford Textbook of Psychiatry, pp 696, 698;
     Companion to Psychiatric Studies, 4th edn, pp 186, 444–445;
     Comprehensive Textbook of Psychiatry, 4th edn, p 1170

9.11 Vulnerability factors greatly increase the risk of depression if a provoking agent is present
Provoking agents
Excess of threatening life events, e.g. bereavement
Chronically stressful situations, e.g. poor housing
Vulnerability factors
Loss of mother before the age of 11
Three or more children, under the age of 14 at home
Lack of a confiding relationship with a husband or other intimate
Lack of a full- or part-time job

> **Ref.** Companion to Psychiatric Studies, 4th edn, p 350;
> Oxford Textbook of Psychiatry, p 206

9.12 i   a. enzyme inhibition
         b. phenytoin toxicity
     ii a. mutual enzyme induction
         b. reduced concentration of both carbamazepine and phenytoin
    iii a. synergism
         b. lithium toxicity
     iv a. enzyme induction
         b. contraceptive failure

> **Ref.** Hallworth M J, Brodie M J 1987 Therapeutic monitoring of phenytoin. Hospital Update 13: 838

9.13 a. More familiar
             Easier to undertand
             Easier to remember
             Easier to use
             Ready prelude to action — e.g. diagnosis may imply treatment
             Less strain on resources of the profession (which is largely innumerate)
         b. Convey more information since finer distinctions are possible
             More flexible — they can easily be converted into any number of categories, and back again
             Do not imply the presence of unproven qualitative differences between members of different subpopulations
             Do not impose boundaries where none may exist
             Do not distort the observer's perception of individuals lying near the boundary between adjacent categories

> **Ref.** Companion to Psychiatric Studies, 4th edn, pp 221–222

9.14 **Placebo effect** — any treatment produces beneficial results if taken or given with enough faith and enthusiasm
Hawthorne effect — better response from subjects who believe an interest is being taken in them
Natural remission — the condition being studied remits naturally and if this is likely to occur to any great extent before the time when the trial is to be completed then the treatment results may be confused with the natural response
Practice effect — the performance of the subject may change as successive assessments are carried out and the subject and experimenter become used to the procedure

Ref. Companion to Psychiatric Studies, 2nd edn, p 232

9.15 Delta (slowest)
Theta
Alpha
Beta
a. Benzodiazepines
    Barbiturates
b. Neuroleptics
    Tricyclic antidepressants

Ref. Comprehensive Textbook of Psychiatry, 4th edn, pp 90, 97

9.16 The principle of family studies involves comparison of the rates of illness in the first- and second-degree relatives of probands. First-degree relatives, e.g. parents, share on average 50% of the genes of the proband, whilst second-degree relatives, e.g. grandparents, share on average 25%. Therefore, for a genetic disorder there should be, on average, greater similarity between a proband and his or her close relatives, than between people drawn from the population at large
Problems and solutions
Shared environment can lead to resemblance between relatives. **Solution** — twin studies and adoption studies
Remitting and relapsing nature of disorders and variable age of onset. **Solution** — compare relatives according to whether or not they have had an illness in their entire life — lifetime incidence
Some relatives may be too young to be affected by a given condition at the time of a study, and others may only have lived through part of the age of risk. **Solution** — correct for age, e.g. Weinberg's method
(Give any two)

Ref. Companion to Psychiatric Studies, 4th edn, 165

9.17 **a.** Eysenck Personality Inventory
Minnesota Multiphasic Personality Inventory
 b. Thematic Apperception Test
Rorschach Inkblot Test

Ref. Comprehensive Textbook of Psychiatry, 4th edn, pp 514–529;
Companion to Psychiatric Studies 4th edn, pp 324, 408–409

9.18 Supersensitivity is said to occur when the response to an
agonist is greater than the previously established maximum
response. It helps maintain synaptic function when the receptor
density and/or amount of neurotransmitter is reduced
Evidence
Tardive dyskinesia may be precipitated by stopping neuroleptic
treatment suddenly
Tardive dyskinesia is made worse by stopping neuroleptic
treatment suddenly
Tardive dyskinesia is made worse by L-dopa
Increasing the amount of neuroleptic treatment may lead to a
temporary improvement

Ref. Companion to Psychiatric Studies, 4th edn, pp 113–114, 120;
The Scientific Basis of Psychiatry, pp 233–234

9.19 **a.** The rate of development of new cases in a given population
over a given period of time
 b. The proportion of a given population which has a given
disorder at a defined period of time
 c. [The incidence rate with a risk factor] minus [the incidence
rate without the risk factor]

Ref. Comprehensive Textbook of Psychiatry, 4th edn, pp 301, 303

9.20 It is the maximum correlation between a dependent variable
and multiple non-random independent variables as determined
by a least-squares criterion
Assumptions include
The dependent variable is normally distributed
The independent variables are non-random, fixed values
Random errors in the model are normally distributed
Random errors in the model have a mean of zero
(Give any three)

Ref. Comprehensive Textbook of Psychiatry, 4th edn, pp 334–335

Reference List

American Psychiatric Association 1987 Diagnostic and statistical manual of mental disorders, Third Edition — Revised (DSM-111-R). American Psychiatric Association, Washington, DC

Andrews J G, Tennant C 1978 Life event stress and psychiatric illness. Psychological Medicine 8: 545–549

Atkinson R C, Atkinson R C, Hilgard E R 1983 Introduction to psychology, 8th edition. Harcourt Brace Jovanovich, San Diego

Barraclough B M, Mitchell-Heggs N A 1978 Use of neurosurgery for psychological disorder in the British Isles during 1974–6. British Medical Journal ii: 1591–1593

Bebbington P 1987 John Connolly. In: Thompson C (ed) The originals of modern psychiatry. Wiley, Chichester

Berrios G E 1987 Outcome prediction and treatment response in schizophrenia. Practical Reviews in Psychiatry, Series 2, 3: 7–9

Berrios G E, Dowson J H (eds) 1983 Treatment and management in adult psychiatry. Bailliere Tindall, London

Bondy P, Rosenberg L E (eds) 1979 Metabolic control and disease, 8th edition. Saunders, Philadelphia

British Medical Association and the Pharmaceutic Press 1988 British National Formulary, No. 15. British Medical Association and the Pharmaceutical Press, London

Brown G W, Harris T 1978 Social origins of depression. Tavistock, London

Carpenter W T, Strauss J S, Muleh S 1973 Are there pathognomonic symptoms of schizophrenia? An empiric investigation of Schneider's first rank symptoms. Archives of General Psychiatry 28: 847–852

Cerletti U, Bini L 1938 Un nuovo metodo di shokterapia; 'l'elettroshock'. Bulletin Accademia Medica di Roma 64: 136–138

Connolly J 1856 The treatment of the insane without mechanical restraints. Reprinted 1981. State Mutual Books, USA

Cooper J E, Kendell R E, Gurland B J et al 1972 Psychiatric diagnosis in New York and London. Maudsley Monograph No 20. Oxford University Press, London

Dean C, Kendell R E 1981 The symptomatology of puerperal illnesses. British Journal of Psychiatry 139: 128–133

Downey L J, Malkin J C (eds) 1986 Bulimia nervosa — current approaches. Duphar Laboratories Limited, Southampton

Edwards G 1976 Cannabis and the psychiatric position. In: Graham J D P (ed) Cannabis and health. Academic Press, London

Forrest A D, Affleck J W, Zealley A K (eds) 1978 Companion to psychiatric studies, 2nd edition. Churchill Livingstone, Edinburgh

Freeman W, Watts J W 1942 Psychosurgery. Thomas, Springfield, Ill

Frommer E A 1968 Depressive illness in childhood. In: Coppen A, Walk A (eds) Recent developments in affective disorders. Headley Brothers, Kent

Gelder M, Gath D, Mayou R 1983 Oxford textbook of psychiatry. Oxford University Press, Oxford

Goffman E 1968 Asylums. Penguin, London

Graham P, Rutter M 1985 Adolescent disorders. In: Rutter M, Hersov L (eds) Child and adolescent psychiatry: modern approaches, 2nd edition. Blackwell, Oxford

Graham P, Rutter M 1973 Psychiatric disorder in the young adolescent: a follow-up study. Proceedings of the Royal Society of Medicine 66: 1226–1229

Harlow H F, Griffin G 1965 Induced mental and social deficits in rhesus monkeys. In: Osler S F, Cooke R F (eds) The biological basis of mental retardation. John Hopkins University Press, Baltimore

Hift E et al 1960 Results of shock therapy on schizophrenics in childhood. Schweizer Archiv fur Neurologie, Neurochirurgie und Psychiatrie, 86: 256

Kanner L 1943 Autistic disturbance of affective contact. Nervous child 2: 217–250

Kaplan H E, Sadock B J (eds) 1985 Comprehensive textbook of psychiatry, 4th edition. Williams and Wilkins, Baltimore

Kasl S V, Cobb S 1966 Health behaviour, illness behaviour and sick-role behaviour. Archives of Environmental Health 12: 246–266

Kellam A M P 1987 The neuroleptic malignant syndrome, so-called: a survey of the world literature. British Journal of Psychiatry 150: 752–759

Kendell R E, Zealley A K (eds) 1983 Companion to psychiatric studies, 3rd edition. Churchill Livingstone, Edinburgh

Kendell R E, Zealley A K (eds) 1988 Companion to psychiatric studies, 4th edition. Churchill Livingstone, Edinburgh

Kerr A, Snaith P 1986 Contemporary Issues in Schizophrenia. Gaskell

Kral VA 1962 Senescent forgetfulness: benign and malignant. Canadian Medical Association Journal 86: 257–260

Lacey J H, Dolan B M 1988 Bulimia in British Blacks and Asians: a catchment area study. British Journal of Psychiatry 152: 73–79

McGuffin P, Shanks M F, Hodgson R J 1984 The Scientific Principles of Psychopathology. Grune and Stratton, Academic Press, London

Macleod J (ed) 1981 Davidson's principles and practice of medicine, 13th edition. Churchill Livingstone, Edinburgh

Maguire G P, Julier D L, Hawton K E, Bancroft J H J 1974 Psychiatric morbidity and referral on two general medical wards. British Medical Journal i: 269–270

Paykel E S 1978 Contribution of life events to causation of psychiatric illness. Psychological Medicine 8: 245–253

Paykel E S (ed) 1982 Handbook of affective disorders. Churchill Livingstone, Edinburgh

Plant M A 1979 Occupations, drinking-patterns and alcohol-related problems: conclusions from a follow-up study. British Journal of Addiction 74: 267–273

Randall F, Wright F J 1981 Basic sociology, 4th edition. M & E Handbooks, Macdonald and Evans, Plymouth

Reid A H 1982 The psychiatry of mental handicap. Blackwell, Oxford

Roth M 1955 The natural history of mental disorder in old age. Journal of Mental Science 101: 281–301

Rubenstein D, Wayne D 1980 Lecture notes on clinical medicine, 2nd edition. Blackwell Scientific Publications, Oxford

Russell G F M 1979 Bulimia nervosa: an ominous variant of anorexia nervosa. Psychological Medicine 9: 429–448

Russell W R, Smith A 1961 Post-traumatic amnesia in closed head injury. Archives of Neurology 5: 4–17

Rutter M, Chadwick O, Yule W 1976 Adolescent turmoil: fact or fiction. Journal of Child Psychology and Psychiatry 17: 35–56

Rutter M, Cox A, Tupling C, Berger M, Yule W 1975 Attainment and adjustment in two geographical areas I: the prevalence of psychiatric disorder. British Journal of Psychiatry 126: 493–509

Rutter M, Graham P, Birch H G 1970 A neuropsychiatric study of childhood. Clinics in Developmental Medicine No. 35. Spastics International Medical Publications in Association with Heineman Medical Books, London

Rutter M, Shaffer D, Shepherd M 1975 A multiaxial classification of child psychiatric disorders. World Health Organisation, Geneva

Rutter M, Tizard J, Whitmore K (eds) 1970 Education, health and behaviour. Longmans, London

Rutter M, Yule B, Quinton D et al 1975 Attainment and adjustment in two geographical areas III: Some factors accounting for area differences. British Journal of Psychiatry 126: 520–533

Sheldon W H, Steven S S, Tucker W B 1940 The varieties of human physique. Harper, London

Sheldon W H, Steven S S, Tucker W B 1942 The varieties of temperament. Harper, London

Shields J 1980 Genetics and mental development. In: Rutter M (ed) Scientific foundations of developmental psychiatry. Heineman Medical Books, London

Snell R S 1987 Clinical neuroanatomy for medical students, 2nd edition. Little, Brown and Company, Boston

Swinscow T D V 1983 Statistics at square one. British Medical Association, London

Symington N 1986 The analytic experience. Free Association Books, London

Taylor M A, Abrams R 1973 The phenomenology of mania. A new look at some old patients. Archives of General Psychiatry 29: 520–522

Walton J N 1977 Brain's diseases of the nervous system, 8th edition. Oxford University Press, Oxford

Weissman M M, Klerman G L 1977 Sex differences and the

epidemiology of depression. Archives of General Psychiatry 34: 98–110

Weller M (ed) 1983 The Scientific basis of psychiatry. Bailliere Tindall, London

World Health Organization 1978 Mental disorders; glossary and guide to their classification in accordance with the ninth revision of the International Classification of Diseases (ICD-9) World Health Organization, Geneva

Yalom I D 1975 The theory and practice of group psychotherapy, 2nd edition. Basic Books, New York